NOODLES FOR DUMBBELLS

Water Exercise, Weight Management & More

by

JANNA LOWELL

PublishAmerica
Baltimore

First printing

Hardcover 9781630004156
Softcover 9781462664429
PUBLISHED BY PUBLISHAMERICA, LLLP
www.publishamerica.com
Baltimore

Printed in the United States of America

NOODLES
FOR DUMBBELLS

Water Exercise, Weight Management & More

Contents

PREFACE

It was my good fortune to come into the water exercise experience professionally twenty-some years ago when being in the right place, at the right time; I landed many featured spots on network and cable TV. It seemed that the media, in quest of the latest commercial video opportunity, were eager to demonstrate that water aerobics was becoming something more than the refuge of the 'silver tsunami' of retiring Americans treating their aches and pains. Once, I fell asleep with the TV on and awakened much later that night to *ACCESS* or *HARD COPY* rerunning a clip; it was my own voice that startled me to attention as my aquatics class paraded before my eyes. It was the kind of wide-awake-nightmare that made me rethink holding classes in the noonday sun...

When I came on the scene, water exercise was exploding as a sports training method for elite athletes and as an ideal rehabilitation method for patients recovering from hip and knee replacements as well as accident injuries. There are several terrific books on the market that address these readers needs very well, having been authored and co-authored by therapists and doctors. They offer specific isolated exercises for strengthening and/ or rehabilitating various joints and muscles as well as the necessary precautions.

My focus as a group exercise instructor has been on meeting the needs of the average class participant from post rehab to cross training athletes, gorgeous models to famous actors, newly pregnant athletic young woman and their husbands as well as the soon to be grandparents. Generally, 'my people' are battling encroaching middle-aged metabolic breakdown and the weight gain that frequently accompanies it. Sometimes it's just the annoying and seemingly inevitable thickening of the waistline or the inability to continue on with a previous hi intensity exercise program. Whether it be the pounds that are difficult to shed after pregnancy, or the pounds that add up after a sports or accident injury, there is a general consensus that it is difficult to get them off and keep them off. In most cases, when new members come participate in my classes, it is with little knowledge or understanding of the benefits to be had in water other than pain relief and no understanding of the real opportunity. Frequently, it's with desperation to *do something* that you show up.

During these years that I have been training, the obesity epidemic has turned our country into a population that is predominantly overweight and frightfully obese in numbers. While America has been the number one leader in many things, this is our most undesirable 'win'. Even our military is 'up in arms' over the lack of qualified applicants!

Having trained extensively in nutrition before it was embraced by medical schools, it has been a subject of constant fascination for me and one that I cannot help but apply to my students' success or failure at weight management.

Consequently, my main purpose here is to address aquatic exercise as a really fun and effective means to stimulate your metabolism while also presenting the most promising and useful new information on weight management. My objective is to deliver both the motivation, and the means. My workout techniques are explained and demonstrated, as much as possible, in what I hope is a more intuitive approach than what we generally see in books. It is more difficult than I'd imagined writing about exercise and equally challenging to try and convey movement in a still picture drawing.

I do know that many of you grew up watching exercise videos featuring the likes of Jane Fonda, *THE FIRM* and other more recent pro's that've delivered a wide variety of low impact steps from dance to fitness. These are the moves I draw upon in these pages. Such things as jumping jacks and lunges take on many new variations when we add the properties that are unique to water. They become fun in ways that they never could on land.

I have tried to put these exercises and routines together in such a way that most anyone can participate to some extent, keeping in mind your physical limitations. My bigger challenge is to push more of you towards your aerobic threshold where you will get the maximum metabolic boost from your workout. That requires moving quickly from one exercise to the next, building in intensity, utilizing interval training and even explosive plyometric moves whenever possible in order to meet the necessary criteria.

On that score, this should serve as an excellent workbook for those who do take class with me. I have tried to answer your most frequent and relevant questions and give you access to my accumulated knowledge. Sometimes, we don't know what questions to ask, we are busy leading our lives and unaware that new solutions are available. There was a glut of new information just hitting the market as I began writing this book and I have attempted to include some mention of everything I think might be worthy of further investigation or helpful in terms of meeting your goals and achieving lasting results.

If you pick up this book in hard copy or digitally in some remote corner of the world, you may yet find classes and instructors who are AEA certified. If not, please don't let that deter you. It may require a learning curve before you have combination moves and transitions down that allow for a rapid pace, but you can always pick the pace up by adding drills. Above all, try to have a good time and don't worry too much about getting it right. If any given exercise is painful (even in triggering old pains), that is a good indication that it's not the right move for you; at least, not yet. Try again when you've gotten stronger and you may be pleasantly surprised.

Please note that this book is not intended to provide medical advice- neither the author, nor publisher take responsibility for any possible consequences for any treatment, procedure, exercise, dietary modification, action or application of medication which results from reading or following the information contained in this book. The publication of this information does not constitute the practice of medicine and does not replace the advice of your physician or health care provider. Before undertaking any course of treatment, the reader must seek the advice of their physician.

Additionally, please note that I am not a representative of any company selling any product that is mentioned, discussed or recommended in these pages. I do not benefit in any monetary capacity by advocating for them... though in many cases, I would love to!

ACKNOWLEDGEMENTS

With gratitude to Dr. Barbara Ann Roth: long before she was a doctor, she was a much beloved aerobics instructor who led me straight to my life in the swimming pool. To Toni Brown and Pat Soley for keeping me employed at the most beautiful swimming pool in town. To Marcella Jennings for demonstrating that an occasional Martini should perhaps be listed as a 'wellness' cocktail. To Alice and Ed Colton, Lucien and Jerry Aroesty for proving that couples do it consistently.

To my sister Darlene, for mid-wifing the birth of this 'baby', and my sister Linda; your enthusiasm, and desire to see me succeed have kept me going. To my niece Sherah, for taking great pictures and encouraging her auntie to complete this adventure on paper. To my Mom, for all your blessings. To Moses Shenassa and Ali Ghazi, my gratitude for your help and patience.

To Jennifer Brown for being willing to 'share', to Penelope Gillette for confirming that book-worthy material lurks in these pages, to Carol Rosenstein for your encouragement, to Erica Lamrell and Martin Morris for giving me constructive criticism when it matters most. To Anita Dymont, Harriet Rolnick, Jilliene Bolker, Nazy Mohajer, and Mooluch Molayem for your on-going support. To Joanne, Marcy, Sica, Scarlet, Elise, Isabella, Brandy, Sheila, Lorna, Beny, Manaz, Cynthia, Gina, Ora, Mitra, Adrianna, Anita, Dayan, Parvin, Michael, Nina, Kathy, Dianne, Sue, Jan, and all the 'regulars' who make life interesting, I thank you!

FOREWORD

A few years ago, Ms. Lowell came into my office for a physical that caused quite a bit of commotion with my staff. When attempting to begin the standard 'stress test' on Janna, they came running to get me, extremely concerned over her slow pulse. I had to instruct my staff- "Calm down! What you are observing, ladies, is something we seldom see in this office; an extremely *fit* person!"

Over the past twenty years, the subject of obesity has been discussed widely in both the lay and medical press. Even a T.V. show- *THE BIGGEST LOSER* has made obesity a primary theme. Yet, no significant progress has been made in combating this epidemic.

Obesity contributes to cardiovascular disease, joint disease, and even psychological problems. No one has the magic cure. However, two things are most important, eating properly, and exercise. For many people, running or even brisk walking outside as well as exercising on a treadmill or elliptical is very difficult to impossible because of neuromuscular and/ or arthritic problems. This is where water aerobics plays a great role in allowing people with these issues to increase their metabolism and burn calories without causing additional pain and injury to themselves. However, it's quite possible that many of you, like me, have observed a rather lame looking class at your local gym, and walked away unimpressed and uninspired to give it a try.

Ms. Lowell, an eminently qualified water aerobics instructor, does an excellent job of explaining how you can achieve an optimal cardiovascular workout to burn more calories and strengthen the core musculature of the trunk utilizing the special properties unique to a water environment. Additionally, her life long study of nutrition allows her to offer up some of the most current thinking on dietary concerns that may have been a roadblock to achieving or maintaining your weight management goals. For those of you who cannot exercise 'on land' as well as the fitness buff looking for variety, this book is a must read.

Dr. Allan Cohan, September 2012

Pharma' as it's main course of action... and it's no wonder!

As a fitness professional with more than thirty years experience in diet and exercise, I have seen over and over again how difficult it is for the average 'dumbbell' who has become set in their ways to make real and lasting changes in their lifestyle. I know that such changes are within your reach. I see it happening daily as I participate in the process with those who come to me as clients, as participants in my classes. Unfortunately, so many people wait until they have a dire medical prognosis, until they are literally filled with fear before they consider the options that are readily available to them. It is my objective, in these pages, to simplify the process for you. I want to help you take a quantum leap out of your belief system. It has been demonstrated that it takes twenty-one days to break a bad habit. The reverse may well be true. By choosing to implement new and better habits, by using your 'noodle'... you can slowly become the person that you might prefer to be. After all is said and done, your health and fitness is no joke!

In these pages, it is my heartfelt desire to help you benefit from my experiences as an 'accidental athlete'. The habits that I have developed out of necessity are habits that now constitute the basis for the good health and longevity which (I hope you agree!) I appear to be enjoying. I am including chapters that can help you with diet, but truthfully, I do not believe in a 'diet' per say or even 'dieting'. I am fond of 'cleansing my system' when I've been a little naughty... it actually feels good to cleanse when you are experiencing the negative consequences of poor food choices. Those poor food choices will have a very real impact on your energy, on your vitality, on your sexuality, usually, on the very next day...just like the hangover you experience from alcoholic beverages.

When you bring your system into balance, it is no big deal making corrections when you've slipped up and veered off course for a day. Perhaps I shouldn't even call it 'slipping up' because I generally plan my indulgences when I know that I am attending a celebration or event where there will be an abundance of delicious food and drink. If you get your workouts in regularly before that event and tweak your consumption just a little before and after - you do not necessarily have to suffer negative consequences.

This may sound like magical thinking to many of you fighting overweight and to the 'underlean' who are not obviously fat but suffering from all the metabolic conditions that lead to what has now been termed 'diabesity'. One in four 'skinny' people is now considered to be 'MONW' or metabolically obese, normal weight. These underlean yet overfat individuals lack muscle mass and tend towards belly fat putting them at *twice* the risk of death as the so-called 'fit and fat' individual, according to *THE JOURNAL OF THE AMERICAN MEDICAL ASSOCIATION* or AMA. While sixty-eight percent of America is overweight, 'diabesity' describes the metabolic breakdown that falls somewhere between prediabetic and type 2 diabetes. Meanwhile, doctors are also seeing more cases of type 1 diabetes appearing in adults. According to the CDC, childhood obesity has tripled in the past thirty years, but because symptoms of diabetes may be lacking, only a blood test to measure glucose metabolism will give an accurate diagnosis. As diabetes is a life-long disease that must be managed through diet, exercise, and medication, it puts a very real emotional and financial stress on the family as the diabetic individual will spend $4,100 or more on annual medical costs. In fact, it is estimated that two hundred billion dollars a year is now spent on such obesity related expenses.

It seems to me that the biggest mistake many overweight people make is in deciding somehow that their 'ideal' weight is so far removed from their current weight that nothing short of Herculean efforts or surgical intervention will help. It is a self-defeating attitude that stands in the way of your improved health and appearance, and it generally prevents you from getting started. I deal with people every day who confide in me- "I know that I have to lose forty pounds!" I try to get them to see that losing ten pounds in the next few months is doable. Exercising will also convert some of that stored fat into muscle. You can lose inches without losing pounds. There is such a thing as a 'set point' which is a term you are familiar with if you are a yo yo dieter; losing and gaining that same amount over and over. This is the weight that your body will slowly go back to unless you try something different to shake up the process. The single factor that is indicated over and over in successful long-term weight loss is *exercise*, regular, consistent exercise.

Before going any further, my experience has also proven to me just how difficult it is for many people to tell their family and friends, clients or bosses that they have set aside a certain hour daily for exercise. 'Exercise and the gym' have connotations that allow for argument, that allow for ridicule! Sometimes these people have an agenda of their own that will interfere with yours. It's so easy for them to make you feel guilty... to make you feel that something else is more important. My advice: Don't tell them that you're going to workout, tell them instead that you've got therapy scheduled in that time slot (it will prove to be therapeutic!) or perhaps, better yet, don't pick up the phone. You must give yourself permission! Decide that there is nothing more important than your health and happiness. Decide that everyone else will benefit from your increased health and happiness. Decide to begin now!

heat capacity of any substance on Earth, which means it plays a powerful role in regulating our planets temperature. All that and yet ninety-eight percent of the surface water on our planet is salt water, leaving only one percent fresh water that is available for human consumption, meaning it will certainly take on increasing political significance in the coming years.

In training to become a certified aquatics instructor, we covered the physical laws as they are applied to the aquatic environment. I studied "how the water works" so that I could more effectively teach you "how to work the water." Everybody knows through first hand experience that we react differently to movement in water as compared to those same movements on land. But wait, I may be wrong... many people have drowned performing movements that don't work in the water! Interestingly, babies seem to have an instinct here- perhaps a throwback to those months spent floating in amniotic fluids. We get older and we loose those instincts, becoming fearful, or else, we become good swimmers.

Taking a vertical approach to exercise in water can be a welcome departure from the repetitive motion that constitutes swimming. It opens a world of joyful new possibilities! Jump into the water and it seems that there's much less gravity at work. Actually, the force of gravity is the same in water as it is on land. What's happening really is that an object placed in water will displace an amount of water *equal* to its volume. That displaced water then pushes up on the object with a force *equal* to the force of gravity. In other words, the waters **buoyancy** operates *against* the force of gravity. However, if the objects density is less than the density of water... guess what? It floats!

Once, I had an obese lady attend my class on a day when I happened to be teaching from the side of the pool. I watched sympathetically as she flailed about in the water with no apparent ability to control her movements. I was thinking that she lacked core strength and range of motion as well as muscle mass, all of which would improve considerably with regular attendance. At the end of class, she struggled out of the pool and mustered what strength she had to come tell me face to face that my class was useless, a terrible workout... she felt nothing! My mentor at the time informed me that this is what we call a floater. A floater among the unfit... floating away from my class never to return (sometimes that's OK with me!).

At a recent Fourth of July party, I was dismayed when a fellow guest mentioned that he would be interested in aquatic exercise when he didn't see a bunch of overweight women bobbing about in the pool. Sadly for him, but fortunately for these women, there is great relief to be found in having a bit of exercise where your joints won't be aching quite so much, where you will experience your body weight at fifty to ninety percent less than your accustomed land weight, and where you may have a greater ability to move with ease. However, just like our fellow in question, many of the reasonably fit people I encounter are quick to make assumptions about vertical exercise being wimpy and so they fail to see the incredible opportunity.

Swimming, which always has a studly reputation, is all about overcoming and *minimizing* drag forces in order to increase ones speed in what is often a repetitive range of motion. Shaving of the legs and chest, investing in the newest swimwear designed to help us mimic fish, whatever it takes to make us more competitive. Vertical exercise, on the other hand, is completely the opposite; an athletically challenging session is one where you *maximize* the drag forces and put them to work strengthening your core as well as every major muscle group and lot's of fun, effective equipment is marketed to that end. I would say that synchronized swimming is the lovely, athletic result of merging both sets of skills.

Many new instructors and trainers coming from a swim background have problems, initially, in manipulating the unique properties that make vertical exercise so effective and exclusive to water. I know that I always need to jump in and try something new *myself* before I can effectively present it to a class. It's enough of a challenge for an instructor having people of all fitness levels attending one class. At most facilities, I am cueing to the fittest population to push them toward their maximum effort while also cueing to participants who are struggling with recovery from surgery or dealing with long or short term disabilities as well as arthritic conditions. Many of this later group have strict orders from their doctors and know what they cannot/ should not be doing.

It's so important to open up a dialogue with new class participants. When people don't know and don't appear to be particularly athletic, it's always good advice to take it easy in the beginning. I'm fond of saying that even if you do just the simplest steps, standing in the middle of my "Making Waves" class with the participants working hard nearby, the water will make you feel better and slowly get stronger. The movement of the class in its entirety will cause the liquid to swirl about your body, massaging your muscles and facilitating lymphatic drainage. If, at first, the water seems a little too cool, it will numb your aches and pains and leave you feeling invigorated.

Also, it makes sense that the deeper one goes into the water; the more opportunity exists for a decrease in weight bearing forces on all joints and the discs of the spine as well.

Rehabilitation in water became popular because buoyancy enables the weakened area of the body to be supported allowing for an easier and less painful range of motion. Also, an even **hydrostatic pressure**, which increases with the depth of water, helps to eliminate swelling and circulatory problems. This pressure causes the static fluid buildup around injured, painful joints to move upward toward the heart. In my studies, I found it interesting that one of the reasons aquatic exercise is often recommended for patients with a heart history is that the heart rate tends to stay thirteen to seventeen points lower in water than it will on land with the same exertion; resulting in a safer workout. In researching this book, I've come to understand that most experts believe the "mystery" is due to this phenomenon of hydrostatic pressure.

Because buoyancy is resistive and supportive and the hydrostatic pressure is equal on submerged body parts, water is a very safe environment to regain strength, endurance, balance, and flexibility. But don't wait for injuries or disease to take your fitness training to the pool! These same characteristics are now bringing most professional athletes to the water in a well-considered plan to improve their performance and the length of their career in the bargain. After twenty years of aquatic exercise participation, I now value it more than ever. I don't believe I would still be teaching my current load of spinning and sculpting classes or running the occasional 5K race if not for the tremendous benefits that come with my water workouts.

I like to finish my aquatic "Making Waves" classes with some standing yoga poses... poses where we focus on our breathing, balance—on directing the blood flow to the base of the spine. I can't help but dream that someday soon, I may be able to lead my entire class in a guided meditation where we express our love and appreciation to the precious molecules of H2O in our beautiful pool. Imagine if an entire swimming pool was filled with molecules that look like the pictures of Dr. Masaru Emoto's water exposed to love and appreciation. I can't help but wonder what the benefits would be ... could our injuries heal faster... could we feel even happier, healthier, focused, and possibly (dare I say?) care-free as we leave the club and re-enter the stress inducing traffic of Los Angeles? Yes! This is, of course, a La La thought for La La Land...but what if it works?

CONFESSIONS OF AN ACCIDENTAL ATHLETE

"The only way to keep your health is to eat what you don't want, drink what you don't like, and do what you'd rather not."
~ Mark Twain

"We are born naked, wet, and hungry.
Then things get worse."
~ Unknown

This chapter is perhaps completely unnecessary to some readers who want to get started right away with what will be more personally relevant material. Please feel free to skip over this and come back later if and when you may be in a more leisurely frame of mind. My journey as a middle-aged female athlete will not be of interest to everyone. After I pitched this 'expert' book to my generous publisher and was enthusiastically accepted, this was the first content material to make it's way to a blank sheet of paper. I include it still because I hope it will speak to some of you who maybe feel a bit stuck in your life. Some of you who feel unable to make your health and fitness the priority you know it needs to be. Somewhere between the power of the dreams, both night and day, that drive our desires and the reality of bills coming due, of care-taking for loved ones, there are the *habits* that get us through our daily grind. Habits can change!

My very first job in what has become known as "The Fitness Industry" came about accidentally when I was invited by the founders to work for what is now one of the largest gym franchises in the country. They were family friends of my future husband. I soon found myself bored out of my mind, depressed, and gaining weight. My job in their sales department demanded that I spend countless (or worse; all too countable!) hours in a freezing, air conditioned, white shag carpeted; hospital white walled, little box of a room. Here I worked my 'shpiel' on innocent victims while the boss listened in on an intercom. My well-rehearsed rap was for all the attractive young women they sent my way. It was my duty to inform them, in our little snowstorm oasis of "privacy", that they would soon be spreading at the hips—boobs drifting towards their knees, chicken wings flapping in the breeze. They would be losing their looks and losing their marketability. If the ring were on the finger... they would be losing the guy! All of this monitored and evaluated by the boss.

It was ironic when I had that same boss commenting on my figure "So fabulous for you that you've managed to retain it..." I was nineteen, I thought he was kidding, but his expression was serious! I'd had many teen years of stuffing cold pizza or left over spaghetti and a cola down my gut for breakfast. Fortunately, I liked dance classes. Five years of Hula and Tahitian Dancing to please my Mother (she was concerned that I might not grow up to be sexy), and eventually Ballet and Modern Dance to please myself. The public schools mandatory gym classes in those smelly old bloomers and the good genes I've been blessed with had saved me to this point.

I was flattered to be cast in a commercial campaign for the company where I was working this particularly boring sales job. I was featured as an instructor showing members how to adjust their stationary bike. It was fun to see my picture in print in all the papers. And even though I didn't care for their white polyester uniform, I couldn't help thinking that I would prefer demonstrating the bike in real life over the psychological mine fields I was tripping in my little white office.

Meanwhile, I noticed that the most successful woman in this company roared up to a very visible parking space in a fancy new sports car each morning, then lit up a cigarette and downed the cup of coffee that began fueling her onslaught upon an unsuspecting public. Lighting another cigarette fifteen minutes later would help her leave the Duncan Donuts box untouched as she passed the employee lounge area and entered her own freezing white domain.

When, after three months or so at this torturous job, I presented the boss with a plan for my imminent departure, all he could say was, "Husband objection! He doesn't like you working these long hours, huh?" *Husband* objection it was... whatever!

People talk about finding their 'sweet spot' in life... how we should follow our hearts, our passion, and eventually, that will lead to abundance, to prosperity in our 'right' livelihood. Well, I've followed my dreams and come up short handed and frustrated but for that 'sweet spot', which must be all the hours of all the days when I've enjoyed the pleasures of aquatic exercise in a beautiful salt water swimming pool. As fate would have it, I have spent many hours of the last twenty years teaching exercise in the water... all too often wondering what it is that I am doing or going to do in my life. In other words, feeling sorry for myself! Meanwhile, the act of getting to the pool each morning and having the multiple benefits of the work as well as the camaraderie of the fascinating individuals who join me has been an incredible blessing. There's that, and it pays the rent... only just!

People don't often realize that the fitness industry (in Los Angeles, at least) is incredibly competitive. All the hard bodied actors waiting to be discovered in film and TV use it as a kind of leverage. An out of work performer with a daily gym habit will frequently train you for less wages as it just doesn't occur to their belief system that they might still be a professional trainer five or ten years down the road.

If you're good at training, the TV shows will come after you with the pitch that you'll get lots of new clients due to the exposure they provide you, because (with few exceptions) they won't be offering compensation either. But, it does look good on the resume! Never mind the Gary 'Abusey', or that Victoria Jackson only wants to show off her handstands. Anna Nicole Smith was a pleasant surprise; so funny. I want whatever she was taking! But seriously, so sad to realize 'on set' that her performances weren't really comedy... rather a pharmaceutically pain free descent into what might otherwise have been her very public humiliation. She had ballooned up in weight but I still I think she would dry hump any living creature, male or female, just to get a laugh. Now, if I could have coached the calisthenics required for the simulated sex acts which she was fond of enacting, (pizza delivery boys, neighbors husband with neighbors wife watching... on and on... and thankfully, fully clothed!) then we might have whipped her into shape.

As I begin writing today, I notice on my wonderful Maynard Astrological Calendar that the planet Neptune, named after the Olympian god of the seas, has moved into direct motion in the Heavens above signaling an auspicious moment to begin this adventure. Neptune is my ruling planet as I am a Pisces woman with minimal earth emphasis in my birth chart. "Looney tunes" some might say ... "A casualty of La La Land" my family must often have commiserated in thinking. We Pisces are not, generally speaking, a practical tribe. Pisces Albert Einstein even had difficulty tying his own shoe laces, according to his nephew, the late Robert Einstein (Robert was a former radiologist who loved to tell his wife we would be down at the pool doing his prescribed routine while begging me to ignore his nasty skin lesions, and allow him the luxury of a sunbathe. Given his eighty-six years of age, and obvious childlike delight in sunshine—who was I to argue?)

I had a near to drowning incident as a young girl entering puberty when my prankster cousins were up from Panama to visit family. Their father was an ambassador and his sister, Santina, was my grandmother (oldest of twelve children!). She had a lovely little shoreline property on the Severn River right off the Chesapeake Bay. Dangerous snakes lurked among the wild blackberries that rose above the sandy dunes and jellyfish competed with the crabs in our rustically charming bit of shore. I remember this well because I so loved to take a pail and climb up the dunes savoring the taste of warm berries fully ripened by the sun. One time my Mother joined me, certainly wanting my company, as she needed to pee. While crouching in the bushes, a snake slithered out and shocked us both as I fumbled to attack it and my mom scrambled out of her crouched position and into her clothes. She must have been menstruating because I got my first lesson on the birds and the bees. My Mom was then studying Freud and wanted to be certain that I shared any future dreams I might have about snakes with her.

Now, my fathers mother, my Mema/ Santina was a great Italian cook as well as a hot looker- but dignified, of course! Her picnics were amazing ... always fried chicken and Italian style potato salad with bits of green pimento olive, sour cream and olive oil. The greens from her garden and the cold Clammer custard pudding must have been particularly delicious that day because the adults were completely oblivious to what was happening just a few feet away. The little bastards from Panama were getting their thrills first by shoving some stinging jelly fish down my swimsuit. Then, their real fun began as they pushed me down under the sandy water - over and over, again and again- 'til my lungs were bursting and my throat was raw from sand.

Oddly enough, some years earlier, at the age of four or five, I'd had a very disturbing recurring dream (sorry, no snakes!). I awakened in the early hours of the morning every single night, landing with a thud on the bedroom floor, my sheet wound tightly like a shroud about my sweaty little body. Tossing and turning as the ship of my dreams went down in a terrible storm at sea. When these horrible nightmares were first beginning, I'd cry until Mommy came to carry me back to my parent's bed and comfort the shivers away.

Eventually, it was my psychic cat Billy who cured me of my nightly trauma by licking my tears away. Billy would disappear for a month or two sometimes only to return covered in bloody scabs from bird peckings. I loyally stood in our yard one day with a big pile of rocks that I'd gathered, aiming at the cat birds as they swopped down again and again to stab their beaks into Billy's wounds. Later that night, presumably sleeping… I heard the laughter in the other room as my parents imitated my shouting and gesturing at the birds. Just like I'd previously heard Mema and all the relatives laughing (while they thought I was napping). They ridiculed my silly girl notion that "One day I would become President of the United States, I can be anything I want when I grow up! ". Torrential laughter!

My other, maternal grandmother, Marion, (my Meme) had a profound effect on my formative years as well. One memorable meal at her home in Daytona Beach, Florida, featured her husband's catch from the days boating excursion, a gigantic red snapper fish, which she stuffed with a crabmeat filling before baking. Meanwhile, my two sisters and I suffered cold chills and boils popping out all over our blistered little bodies as a result of baking under the 'shade' of a palm tree at the beach. We must have been obnoxious brats that day, because our mom so needed to forget her kids and enjoy a little peace and solitude as we napped under a palm tree… she paid dearly for it that night!

I was really impressed a couple years later when Marion's next custom designed home featured a swimming pool just off the family room and she served a cold fruit soup at luncheon… yes *luncheon*! She was a beautiful waspy woman directly descended from Prudence Lowell who came to America on the Mayflower. Real 'Daughter's of the American Revolution' material! Her best gift to me was a little paperback book called *LIFE, LOVE, AND SEAWEED*. I was fortunate to be made aware at a very young age that food can be healing, that miracles can happen when you keep your mind open... when you look for the miracle and work to create the favorable circumstances where it can happen.

Later, I read Henry Bieler's (often called the father of modern nutrition) famous book *FOOD IS YOUR BEST MEDICINE*. Then, I visited Anne Wigmore's Hippocrate's Health Institute in Boston (founder and grandmama of the raw foods movement) where I learned about wheat grass, sprouts, and retention enemas. I studied Iridology and tissue cleansing with the late Bernard Jensen and I also joined The American Academy of Biological Medicine founded by Dr.Paavo Airola (*HOW TO GET WELL*). I was fascinated by the science of applied kinesiology, and became an instructor for The Touch for Health Foundation. I worked as a nutritionist after my torturous tenure in sales. Unfortunately, I found it discouraging that I would give pep talks and meal plans galore only to find that my clients wanted to blame someone else for their failure to shed those unwanted pounds. That someone had to be the person they'd employed to oversee their diet. Unfortunately for me, I could never oversee what actually went into their mouths and down their gut! I've since learned that I prefer to see my clients burn the calories, and create more muscle mass to speed up their metabolism. There is no argument with inches lost!

Before I end this self-absorbed chapter on my childhood influences, I want to say how fortunate I was to have known both of my great grandmothers. Mema's mother had a many storied townhouse in Washington D.C. with every bit of the yard producing wonderful vegetables and fruits, even a grape arbor for making wine. Sometimes Mema would take me to the farmers market so she could help her mother pack-up her stall at the end of the day. It didn't occur to me, at the time, that my 'great' was a working woman, but otherwise why would she be at the market all day and what did she do with the bountiful excess from her garden?

I confess that questions about my great granny's business were completely driven from my mind by the horrors we passed in the butchers stalls as we made our way to her. The hanging sides of beef, the pig's heads, tongues, and guts displayed lovingly with pride... I could never leave that psychological stage where kids recognize that animals are food and stop thinking about it. It also didn't help my impressionable young mind that this area of town was heavily populated by life's unfortunates, missing limbs and hope, reduced to begging for a handout.

It was also disconcerting that my father's side of my family spoke fluent Italian but apparently (to me) this was done in my presence just so they could make jokes about me. I begged to be included, to learn some Italian, but no way! Now I get it... they wanted me to speak and write well in English. But still, they laughed a lot, talking about me, as their gestures clearly indicated... Of course, I had to try my hand at stand up and comedic acting as an adult because I so wanted to control the laughter that was directed my way, to not feel humiliated by it. To feel powerful as opposed to pathetic.

Speaking of powerful, my 'great' made it to her one-hundredth birthday. Two weeks later, she was shoveling snow from a January blizzard off her walkway when she fell and broke her hip. That was it for her! She had no plans or expectations after being mother of twelve, working woman, one hundred years of age. Check out time...

Now Marion's (Meme's) mother was also quite an experience for me. She lived in a little farmhouse in Virginia where she raised chickens, wrung their necks, plucked them clean of feathers, and served them up with dumplings for dinner. I remember fresh biscuits and gravy, little chicken salad stuffed crème puffs and her wonderful hand cranked ice creams. I also remember how I cried hysterically when my mother forced me to go give her a hug and kiss. Today, we would call my great grandmother Dora 'obese', and I am embarrassed to confess that her size frightened me. It terrified me! Poor Dora suffered with diabetes, as did my father's mother. It didn't stop them from enjoying a long life, but it certainly put a crimp in their style.

In High School I had lofty ambitions for an academic life. Many scholastic honors came my way for painting, for writing, and for math. I daydreamed that I would become an Art Professor... long sabbaticals would be spent painting in the far corners of the globe. Now it was my high school boyfriend who would infuriate me in his insistence that I become a gym teacher... a gym teacher? No way! My destiny was calling...

To this day, people come and tell me of their deep-sea diving adventures, insisting that I should get certified, as I would love swimming with the dolphins. And I would, in theory—in my dreams. However, if you watch me very carefully in the water, you may observe that while I am a good strong swimmer- you will never catch me swimming *willingly* with my head under water! And while I never became a gym teacher, per se, I did become a group exercise instructor. An aspiring comedy actress/ writer with a two hour daily gym routine must find a way to pay the rent when she stops accepting bit parts. "We become the thing we are in life because of what we couldn't be" is a saying I have heard that really seems to apply in my case.

First, I fell into teaching Pilates, as I happened to meet two lovely individuals here in LA who had studied and worked directly with Joseph Pilates in New York. It was always interesting to see the celebrities flocking to my friend's studio and they began to ask me to give them a hand when the studio got very busy. I had a knack for Pilates due to my dance background and my love for yoga. In fact, teaching group Pilates to our gay clientele in West Hollywood inspired my first comedic fitness video, *MATIRA, MISTRESS OF MUSCLE, GODDESS OF INTERPLANETARY DISCIPLINE, WHIPS YOU INTO SHAPE.*

Eventually, I found that too many hours spent in a Pilates studio could also result in a sluggish metabolism for me. That's where the beauty of aquatic exercise first dawned upon my vanity. A solid core based cardio workout where every movement is against the natural resistance of water... It was fun and I was hooked! I also love to teach group cycling and sculpting classes but I must say that without the pool time I would be suffering from the brutalities I enjoy dishing out.

One girlfriend insisted some time ago that it wasn't really fair, "You bought yourself an extra twelve to fifteen years of youth and vitality!" I disagree completely. I disagree because I didn't buy them—I earned them! And, I am most happy to help you discover how you can earn them too. Why sell your soul for the 'knifestyles' of the rich and famous in our ageist contemporary society's battle against 'diabesity' when joyful, affordable solutions are within your reach?

As for the rest of my ambitions... it isn't over yet! Though I may well be 'over' in the kind of business model that exists to this day in Hollywood. I saw an enlightening documentary movie recently called *MISSREPRESENTATION*. The statistics that apply to women working in Hollywood are staggeringly negative... just like the statistics that apply to American women in politics. When I won a hard fought little claim in the Writers Guild age discrimination lawsuit last year I continually joked that "I don't know when the sexual discrimination ended and the age discrimination began". With the kind of strong female role models that exist in my family, it never occurred to me that failure was an option. Perhaps I should have tried harder to understand the laughter that was directed my way. Thank God I have my health, my local farmers markets, and a lovely salt-water swimming pool filled with friends that awaits me tomorrow morning. Now it's time for you to come along, we must prepare you to come jump into the pool with me!

DON'T QUIT REMIXED

When the pounds pile on, as they sometimes may,
When modern life's stressors cause more than dismay,
When the economy's tanked and our debts are high,
And you'd love a good laugh, but really need a cry,
When aches and pains seem here to stay,
Come heal in the water, let's call it play!

Life is tough with its ups and downs,
Sunny smiles becoming frightful frowns,
And many in failure have turned away,
When health and happiness were within reach,
Don't give up, though results come slowly,
Just weeks of effort and you won't feel lowly.

Often the goal is nearer than it seems
In a fit of depression, when hunger screams.
Often the struggling dieter has given in,
Munching fries with soda, forget this getting slim!
And he learned too late as he gained more weight,
Just how close he'd come to feeling really great.

New habits take time yet results are sublime,
Dreams can come true, yes, it's all up to you.
Though you can't be certain how close you are;
Success may be near when it seems afar;
So exercise, you can't just sit and wait-
Come jump in the pool, it's not too late!

~ Janna Lowell

MAKING WAVES: BRING THE HEAT

"My goal has always been to help people
help themselves. Your body is your most priceless
possession; you've got to take care of it!"
~ Jack Lalanne

"Health and a good state of body are above all gold,
and a strong body above infinite wealth."
~Ecclesiasticus 30:15

"Everybody pities the weak, jealousy you have to earn."
~ Arnold Schwarzenegger

WATER EXERCISE PREPARATION

As an enthusiastic advocate of the aquatic revolution, it is my goal in the following **MAKING WAVES** section of this book to help you find your own passion for exercising in the water. I am addressing in these pages the average participant who may come and take a class with me. Frequently, that person has had some exercise experience and is looking for cross training fun. She may be very fit and newly pregnant. He/ She may have some injuries that have made their usual workout too painful and are hopeful that water will provide a means to stay in reasonable shape while healing. Sometimes, this person is dealing with a daunting medical diagnosis of serious consequence. They have been made to understand that their quality of life may be substantially better in the months and years to come if they take their exercise program seriously.

Almost always, whether they mention it or not, all of these people are very concerned that their metabolism may be slowing down and the pounds starting to add up. In every case, they made a smart choice and they have come to the right place. In general, according to the MayoClinic, aquatic aerobics will allow for one-third *more* calories burned per class compared to land based aerobics due to the special properties of water. This results in an approximate caloric expenditure of one hundred forty-five to three hundred eighty calories during a *half* hour session. My class sessions are currently of one hour duration and I lead participants through a ten to fifteen minute WARM-UP period where they are encouraged to assess their readiness for more based on their known limitations as well as how they feel today.

From here, you may leave if the warm-up was enough, or proceed to an empty corner of the pool or stairwell if you have special therapeutic exercises to do. I am not a physical therapist but I am including the titles of several wonderful books at the end of this section that do give therapeutic rehabilitation exercises as well as recommendations for books that offer more specialized and/ or advanced water techniques, should this be of interest to you. Despite my years of training and teaching (or maybe it's because of them!), I find that too much information offered up at once can be intimidating. My focus here is to help you put it all together without letting you lose your initial enthusiasm. To that end, I have simplified my choices, directions, and my explanations in a manner that I hope will allow for a more intuitive understanding and progression for you. You will find the neutral spine illustrated as I mention techniques such as 'pulling your belly button up into your ribs" for the purpose of insuring this neutrality, protecting the spine, and strengthening the core musculature. Also, try the various hand positions to build your awareness of how you can assist or impede movement in water.

After the warm-up, we will move into the SPLASH DANCE phase of class where the emphasis becomes focused on **INTERVAL TRAINING**. To date, all of my research offers the conclusion from experts that weight management can become significantly easier for those fortunate individuals who are able to push themselves to a higher threshold of intensity for these relatively short but repeated efforts that we call intervals.

In Japan, they have specialized in these techniques since the nineteen-nineties calling it the **TABATA TRAINING METHOD.** Dr. Izumi Tabata demonstrated that tremendous fitness gains could be had in as little as four minutes by breaking it down into eight repetitions of twenty seconds. That's eight repetitions of twenty seconds performing the selected exercise at *maximum* effort, followed by a recovery of ten seconds. While low intensity exercise of longer duration may burn more calories during the workout, the higher intensity format results in nine times *more* fat loss benefit for every calorie that's burned while exercising. Apparently, the higher intensity format causes more fat and calories to be burned *post* workout. There are combination sets included here that will give you this opportunity. If you're in shape for this, I suggest you begin by attempting four such intervals in a thirty minute workout and slowly build towards eight or nine in a sixty minute format.

WATER EXERCISE PREPARATION

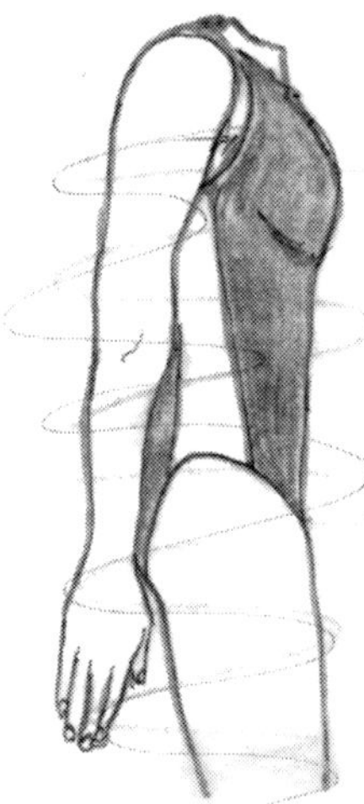

SLICING PALM

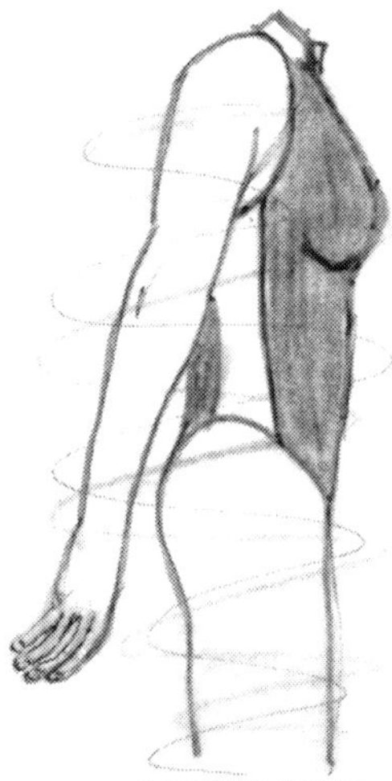

CUPPED PALM

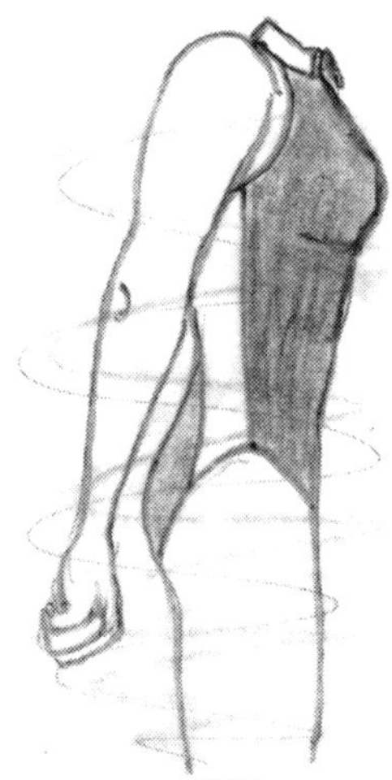

FIST

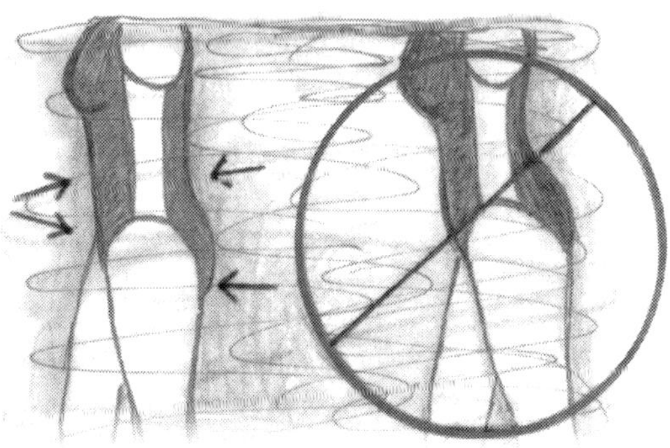

NEUTRAL SPINE

EXPERIANCE
OF GRAVITY
decreased

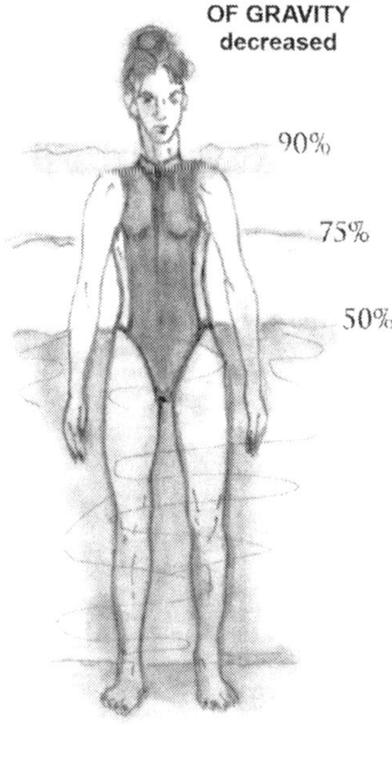

Rx

Doctors Permision: Clarify Your Goals

My plan, you see, is that you discover just how much fun it is to be fit. Be patient here and expect that you will possibly need as many as three months or so of regular practice to get to the *fun* part unless, of course, you are now one of the very fit cross trainers, or a very pregnant woman experiencing immediate relief at the temporary loss of fifty to ninety percent of your body weight. Those of you who previously enjoyed land based high and/ or low impact aerobics classes may also experience instant gratification here.

The USE YOUR NOODLE section then begins as a continuation of the aerobic portion of class but allows for those individuals who may need or prefer to work with no impact to experience challenging intervals. Most of these exercises offer both core emphasis (engaging the stabilizing muscles of the trunk) as well as the benefits of increased circulation, a potentially larger range of motion, and often, a great cellulite massage bonus! We transition with the noodle work into a finishing cool down that makes for a great variety in approaching water exercise.

We complete our training in 'CHILL' NOW with exercises that feature stretching, balance, unloading of the spine, and focused breathing as we prepare to re-enter the gravitational force field that always feels like the new normal as we exit the pool. Additionally, I have included the section GOING DEEP for those who may be persuaded to take the plunge out over your head. This can be incredibly vigorous, but no worries; dumbbells can still use your noodle!

Before getting started, these are some **CONSIDERATIONS:**

1) DOCTOR'S PERMISSION TO EXERCISE: this is a no brainer for those who have been inactive for some time and important for people who have specific issues as well- In fact, you may be reading this book because your doctor suggested water exercise... My suggestion? Discuss and make notes about your objectives with your doctor such as:

a) Weight Loss Goals: is it safe for me to engage in interval training where I will repeatedly approach my maximum heart rate for very short periods followed by recovery? Can wearing a heart rate monitor help me feel more secure and confident in doing so? Can I perform plyometric (propelled up and out of the water) moves or do I have reasons not to? Will losing a few pounds possibly change any of these recommendations? Is my thyroid functioning in the low normal range? If so, can I supplement with a daily drop of Potassium Iodide? (Read more in the chapter SUPPLEMENT THIS!)

b) Special Populations: In conditions such as Parkinson's Disease, MS, arthritis and others, it is generally endurance and range of motion that you want to enhance and preserve. It may be your doctor's recommendation to avoid doing many repetitions of one exercise consecutively. For those seeking to avoid the knee or hip replacement, or other surgery for awhile longer; be certain that you understand what movements are best avoided. Also, you may have prescribed exercises. It will be helpful if you make a copy of them and get it coated with plastic or use a zip lock bag to keep it with you at the pool.

c) The Iron Man Baby Mamma: In recent years, doctors have become fans of the fit mamma and are generally encouraging but be very sure you understand when and how to cut back on intensity as well as duration in your exercise program. You must alter your training to accommodate your bodies changing needs and a heart rate monitor can be instrumental in insuring that you don't over-do. Water, of course, is an ideal environment for taking pressure off that aching back as your pregnancy progresses. In fact, there are many advocates of birthing babies in the water. If this interests you, be certain that you are working with a very experienced professional mid-wife and your doctors full support.

2) CHOOSING A SWIMMING POOL: location, location, location... if it's not nearby, you might find yourself looking for excuses to not go. Many facilities have great pools to choose from at reasonable prices. The local "Y" is often a good option. In some areas here in California, they have more than one type of pool and many different classes to choose from. There are many hotels that will allow swimming pool guests at a reasonable rate, some have classes. Consider the water temperature as well. My preference is for eighty-one or eighty-two degrees. A warmer pool can be uncomfortable and even unhealthy for vigorous exercise. A program designed for Arthritis or featuring Yoga and Pilates or other stretching activities can be a little warmer... perhaps eighty-four to eighty-six degrees. Also, consider whether the pool is chlorinated or salt-water filtration and whether you will be exposed to midday sunshine as sun screen and a visor will be needed (if you can tolerate the sun that you will still be exposed to). If you are a lucky person who can install and maintain your own pool, you might consider a smaller 'endless pool' featuring jets that shoot the water at you. The maintenance will be more affordable and the jets can provide additional resistance and massaging action on your body.

3) YOUR APPAREL: Great deals can be found seasonally at discount stores like Ross and Costco on swimsuits for men and women and sometimes even aquatic exercise shoes but for more reliable year round selections:

a) Women's Wear: I suggest a one-piece swimsuit with racerback or crisscross straps in back so they won't slide down and become annoying. You'll also be more focused on your exercise performance if you don't have to worry about 'the girls' coming out to play, though I've come to believe there are exhibitionists out there who cannot resist giving another kind of performance! If you're self conscious about your tummy, try a 'Miracle Suit', you may not actually look ten pounds thinner, but you won't feel jiggly. For hard to fit sizes and durability, check out www.H2OWear.com.

b) Men's Wear: If you're comfortable in a Speedo, so be it. There are now biker length trunks worn by triathletes that look very comfortable and attractive on a fit body. Consider avoiding the long baggy surfer dude look as the excess fabric will interfere with your range of motion and you will most likely need frequent stops to retie the waist string.

c) Jackets and Vests: The zip-up scuba style jacket or vest is a tremendous investment for those who find the pool temperature chilly and it also helps keep you in the pool year round. Try Kefir, H2OWear or a local scuba diving shop. **TRICK:** shower in warm water before zipping it up, it will then trap that warmth close to your heart.

d) Shoes: Water exercise shoes are recommended but not always necessary. Bad knees, ankles, back and hip issues will benefit from their use. Also, hey are known to provide a little bit of 'drag force' in the water. This can give a cross training fit participant more challenge, as well as the traction which will enable them to perform with more intensity. You can always take a clean pair of washable sneakers to the pool and try them to see if you like the added drag but keep in mind that the high end aquatic shoe has many other advantages in design. Some of the good brands include Avia, Speedo, and Ryka. Many of my class participants favor www.landsend.com for both shoes and swim suits.

e) Moisturizer: Be sure to keep some of your favorite emollient moisturizer in your gym bag and apply liberally post workout shower. You will want to lock the moisture into your skin. I favor a thicker version with some shea butter in the mix, especially in the winter months. While I'm on the subject of skin, this seems as good a place as any to make a special request: please *do not* bring your **perfume** or **aftershave** into the pool with you. Take special care to shower carefully and remove the smells as they will disperse all over the water's surface causing swimmers and class participants to develop animosity toward you, and possibly headaches because they are allergic...

f) Care of Aquatic Apparel: Very important- never leave your wet stuff in a plastic bag sitting in a car parked out in the hot afternoon sun! I have destroyed both swimsuits and shoes this way. **TIP:** spread a towel on the seat or floor and then spread your clothing out so it can dry. Also, beware of the little spin machine, most locker rooms have them but they can easily shred your swimsuit...

4) SPECIAL EQUIPMENT: These days most facilities have an assortment of dumbbells and noodles to choose from. Waist belts are also often available and while they are necessary for most people who intend to do deep water exercise, they are not required for most shallow water work. Sometimes a very bad back or knees can benefit from one in shallow water, but often straddling a noodle will work just as well or better. Other special equipment is available that can make your workout more vigorous and fun, this includes webbed gloves, ankle cuffs, tethers, and other items, which you can find online at www.Aquajogger.com, www.Kiefer.com, and www.Swimoutlet.com. You can request a catalogue from many of these same companies.

5) EAT A SMALL MEAL some time beforehand (usually one and one-half to two hours before is good). For me, this Is critical and I mention it here because far too many people show up to a morning class on an empty stomach not realizing that their blood sugar may be seriously low. While many professionals such as myself have considered this to be a traditionally bad diet plan, new thinking indicates that stored body fat may be effectively burned by exercising with intensity before breakfast. The question is, are you healthy enough to do so? If your doctor agrees that you can try this weight loss technique, you might want to bring a banana or have some other emergency food on hand, just in case. For individuals who tend to run cold, I suggest your morning fuel should include a very small amount of a 'Good Fat' (read more about these in the chapter DIET, WHAT DIET?) For those of you on meds, this could perhaps be left unsaid but I think we can all benefit from a periodic review of our choices. I will also remind you to take an unbreakable **water bottle** if there is no good drinking water available at your pool. Attention to proper hydration is important! Exhaustion is often our only symptom of dehydration which can lead to impairment of thermoregulation and cardiovascular function.

6) CLASSES: I suggest that you have your first water exercise experience in the hands of a properly trained and certified instructor. (For references, phone The Aquatic Exercise Association at 941.486.8600.) This may not be possible or even necessary for the very fit who are cross training but for the special populations it can be an invaluable investment in your wellness and continued participation. In fact, it seems to me that there are many great friendships forged in the water. This is a big motivation to show up on days when you'd rather not. We all know the saying 'misery loves company' is a great testimony to the huge success of group fitness classes in modern America!

GETTING STARTED IN SHALLOW WATER

A THERMAL WARM-UP: This may be sufficient as a stand-alone workout for those who are coming to the pool for the first time and/ or have conditions (pregnancy; if you have not been on a regular exercise program, fibromyalgia, MS, Arthritis, bad knees or back, etc., etc.) that requires careful monitoring. For those who are reasonably fit to very fit, this serves as a signal to your body to prepare for a more vigorous output of energy. It get's the ball rolling, metabolically speaking, and it also gives you an opportunity to assess the condition of your body *today*... if something hurts in the warm-up then you know you must pay extra attention in order to avoid injury. Note that I am assuming you are in a flat bottom lap pool as these exercises performed on a steep slope may create problems. If your pool slopes steeply, you will be better off with deep water training as explained in 'GOING DEEP'.

OPTIONAL EQUIPMENT that you might like to use in your warm-up: why noodles and dumbbells of course! Webbed gloves can be fun as can leg cuffs but I suggest you begin with the basics....

Your warm-up consists of **CROSSING the LENGTH of the POOL** in water that reaches mid-chest, just under the armpits. There are many variations, most of them illustrated here. I recommend most participants try the following for ten minutes or longer-

1) NO ARMS FORWARD: crossing your arms over your chest, relaxed hands resting near the shoulders and **pushing** into the water with the knees slightly bent, head lifted, shoulders down... notice how this engages your core trunk muscles and your sense of balance comes into play-

2) NO ARMS BACKWARD: keeping your arms crossed over your chest, **reverse your direction**, if your knees are not a problem try straightening them as you swing one leg straight backward, then the other... keeping the feet flat as much as possible, you will now notice the musculature of the lower back; an area that many participants want to address, enjoy the massaging action of the water on your back and start to focus your breathing consciously using the exhale portion of a breath to assist as you change to a forward direction-

A THERMAL WARM-UP

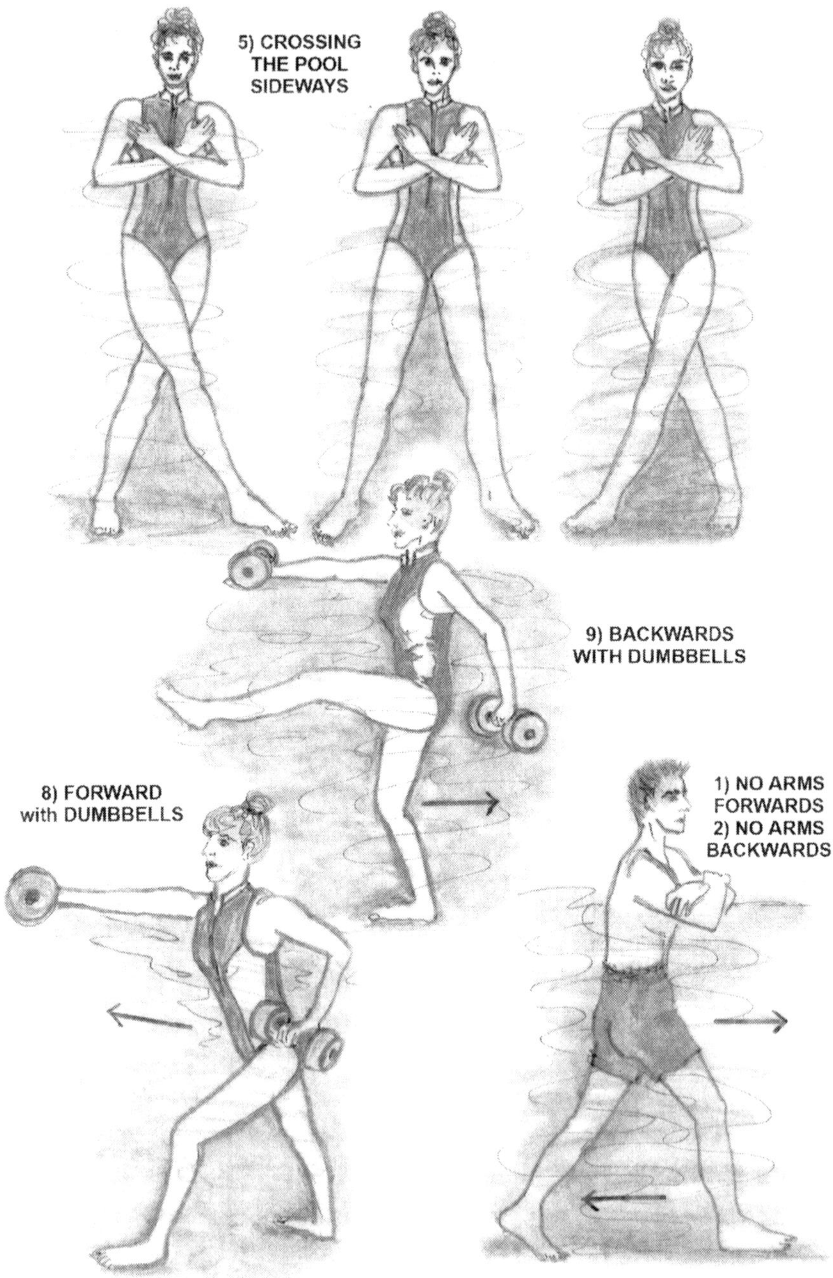
5) CROSSING
THE POOL
SIDEWAYS
9) BACKWARDS
WITH DUMBBELLS
8) FORWARD
with DUMBBELLS
1) NO ARMS
FORWARDS
2) NO ARMS
BACKWARDS

3) SHORTER SETS and **ADDED INTENSITY:** try pushing forward into the resistance of the water for 8 counts and backward for 8 counts, notice how much more challenging the water becomes as you switch directions, how you have to recruit yet more core muscle, now try -4x-forward and -4x- back, it becomes harder still- adding intensity is a matter of flexing those core muscles in the trunk (it may help you to think about pulling the belly button up into the ribs), and increasing the power you apply against the resistance of the water -

4) TIPS: If you feel that you are 'losing control' of your ability to move with intention, if you appear to be 'bobbing about' in the water, most likely the core muscles in your trunk have been neglected, this can occur in a skinny fat or 'underlean' body (lacking muscle mass and prone to similar degenerative metabolic conditions) as well as an overweight or obese body type - In these cases and in the case of the recovering injured, it can be a good idea to begin this set or continue it with the aid of a noodle; try moving forward with the noodle across your chest and under your arms and backward with it across your back (now bending the knees), it will give you both support and added resistance - (please note that this may be enough for your first session if you came to the pool seeking relief from pain... better to do less today and return tomorrow, adding to your individual program as you feel stronger)

5) CROSSING the POOL SIDEWAYS: (Continuing with the arms crossed over your chest or if you need support, a noodle in front of your chest.) Begin with a large step leading with the right leg to your right side and then swing the left leg across the right leg in front, next step right to the side again, then swing the left leg crossing behind the right leg, continue in this manner; swing crossing front, swing crossing back, until you've nearly crossed the pool and then switch directions, most people find that this feels quite wonderful- however, it is contraindicated for hip replacement recipients-

6) FORWARD ADDING ARMS: If you are feeling good and ready for more challenge, we can now try moving forward again and allowing your arms to be pulled backward away from you, notice your shoulder blades being pulled together in back, let your hands relax, keep your shoulders down and your chin dropped slightly- (if your day job has you sitting a lot, this will be good for your back)

7) BACKWARDS WITH ARMS: imagine sitting on a little stool, allow the water to pull your relaxed arms forward, keeping your knees bent, focus on the abdominal contraction by pulling your belly button up into your ribs as you lift those alternating knees up toward the chest- next, go for shorter sets: forward and back -8x-, and then -4x- and added intensity- (you are increasing the resistance of the water by changing your direction and creating more core challenge)-

8) ADDING DUMBBELLS: increase the intensity of the warm-up by moving **forward** with dumbbells resting on the surface of the water, pushing the opposite dumbbell out over the foot in front (knees slightly bent, chest lifted, shoulders down) can you feel how you are engaging the waistline girdle? (pull that belly button up higher and use the exhale to power through) If you have trouble keeping your shoulders down, your dumbbell may be too large, if you are very strong, try pushing them under the surface of the water-

9) BACKWARDS with DUMBBELLS: try alternating kicks backward while still punching the opposite dumbbell out over the foot in front - keep that tummy tight, enjoy the water massage on the back-

10) ROCKING HORSE: going forward again, **(a)** the right knee comes up as you push off the ball of the left foot, **(b)** make a big butterfly with the arms and chest (can be done with or without dumbbells), repeat as desired and **reverse legs**-

11) LITTLE HOPS on the left foot going BACKWARDS: with the right leg lifted up for a stretch, point the toes, flex the heels, circle the ankle, and then reverse the circle with the ankle, meanwhile, circling the dumbbells or the palms of the hands to maintain balance and continue warming-up -

12) REPEAT the ROCKING HORSE: leading with the **left leg** as you move forward again, also **repeating** the little **hops backwards** as you now stretch the **left leg** out, pointing the toes, flexing the heels, circling the ankle, reversing the circles-

13) INTENSITY CROSS: going forward and then backward once more with or without dumbbells, focused on the breathing, power through with the exhale-

A MORE FOCUSED STRETCH: If you decided at some point in the above routine that it was enough for you today, please take an extra moment or two to enjoy the relaxation and recovery benefits of water with a good stretch- If you are fit and eager to accelerate the aerobic portion of your workout, this is an opportunity to assess your readiness for more as well as any areas where you may need to take a more cautious approach-

A THERMAL WARM-UP Continued
& A MORE FOCUSED STRETCH

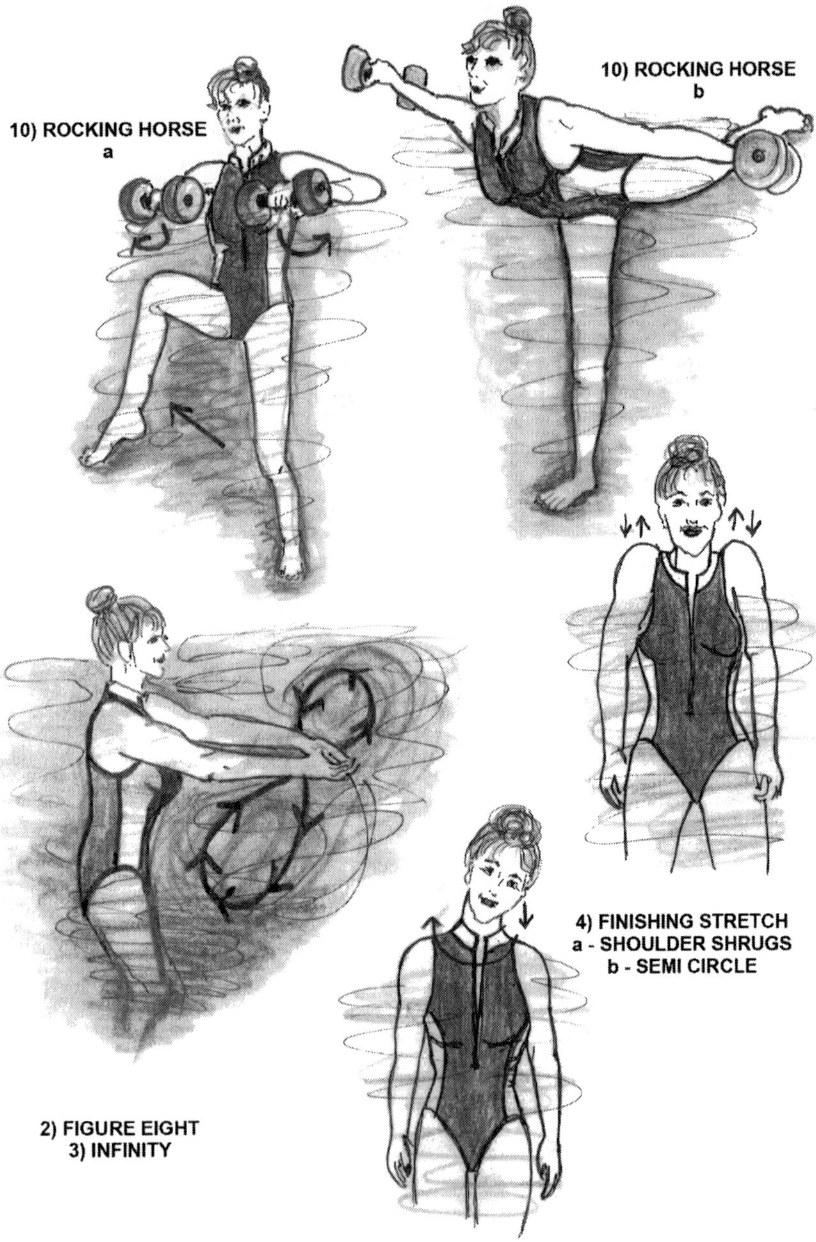

1) CIRCLE: standing in water that reaches mid chest- let your arms go limp, elbows soft, hands completely relaxed, walk in a big **circular motion**, allowing the water to pull your arms back, away from you (keep your knees bent and try to get your shoulders and neck submerged- you cannot get a water massage on body parts that are not in the water!) Now, **REVERSE** your direction-

2) FIGURE EIGHT: keeping the knees slightly bent, feet wide apart and stationary, clasp the thumbs together as you cup the palms of your hands- make a big **figure eight** motion with the arms extended (keeping as much of the shoulders in the water as possible, and dropping your chin a little to follow the hands with your eyes).

3) INFINITY: This is a more strenuous version of the **figure eight** with a bigger range of motion, going from one knee up towards the opposite shoulder and back down towards the knees (this can really carve out the abdominals and strengthen the back (those who have back pain must stick with the easier stretch as above) -really focus on tucking the belly button up into the ribs and using the exhale to power through-

4) FINISHING STRETCH: bringing the feet closer together, **(a)** shrug your shoulders, then **(b)** drop your chin and slowly bring your right ear towards your right shoulder, then left ear towards your left shoulder...next turn your head to the right, then the left and repeat pausing at the point where it just begins to hurt and breathing into the stretch (If you are trying to improve this **range of motion** which is so important for our functional fitness, try a **TRICK:** look away with your eyes only as far as possible while holding the 2nd round of the stretch on each side) Next, reach the long arms together in back, clasp the hands and press up if you're able... finally, stretch those long arms overhead, clasp the thumbs together, and reach to the right, reach to the left, then straight up, lengthening the spine with a last powerful exhale-

MORE HEAT - SOME LIKE IT HOT!: For those who may be dealing with debilitating chronic aches and pains- you might respond well to a thoughtful and systematic use of the jacuzzi. Take an additional ten to fifteen minutes when possible and enjoy those jacuzzi jets. Start with a seated full body position (jacuzzi jets on either side or directly mid-back if you prefer), concentrate on deep breathing and letting go of body tension. Move-on to focus the jets more intently on areas where you experience the most pain. Finish up by opening the palm of each hand comfortably close to the jet, rotate the wrist and reverse it, then each finger and thumb. Finally, (if you're not too ticklish!) see if you can place the bottom of each foot near the jet, it will stimulate your acupressure points as you point the toes, flex the heels, circle the ankles, and reverse the circle. I highly recommend the Arthritis Foundation's 'Hinges and Twinges' program for those who find this helpful. CAUTION: be aware of the water temperature and the length of time if you are unused to the jacuzzi. You can exit the hot water after two minutes and enter a cool pool, repeating this contrasting bath technique a couple times, but always finish up in cool water and apply ice packs to affected areas as heat causes vasodilation (can increase swelling and inflammation) while it is preferable to leave the circulatory system in a state of vasoconstriction. Read more in "CHILL" NOW- MORE CHILL: ICE IS NICE!

MAKING WAVES: SPLASH DANCE

"The word aerobics came about when the gym instructors got together and said 'If we're going to charge ten dollars an hour, we can't call it jumping up and down."
~ Rita Rudner

"I was proud of the waves I had made,
but wondered how many boats I was supposed to rock."
~ Phil Donahue

FOCUSING ON INTENSITY IN WATER AEROBICS

MUSIC SELECTION: I always prefer to teach my classes with music I have specially selected but it becomes even more important when participants are seeking to push themselves to a greater level of fitness. The minor discomfort that you may experience if you're new to aerobics or struggling to shed pounds is greatly offset by some well-loved songs. Also, just by using a planned playlist, you can forget about time and know there will be a motivational song coming up at the time you anticipate a need for inspiration. If this is a do-it-yourself session, I suggest that you enlist a friend or two, or three, when possible. It will help you work harder and longer than you might on your own. For a great selection of downloadable CD's, type in 'POWER MUSIC' at the ITunes store. If you see the beats per minute listed on a CD, most people 'get their groove on' at one hundred twenty-five to one hundred thirty-five bpm in my classes. This kind of continuous beat will enable most reasonably fit people in chest high water to perform sets of four, eight, and sixteen repetitions of a movement using a large range of motion and then allow them to transition vigorously into a different exercise variation. (When I mix my own, I will often go for a faster beat synced to the forty to fifty minute mark for interval training.) For more variety and the most recent releases, go to www.POWERMUSIC.com, or if you want a professional touch, personalize your mix at www.CLICKMIX.com. You can also look at www.DYNAMIXMUSIC.com, www.MUSCLEMIXES.com, and www.YESFITNESSMUSIC.com for motivating CD's.

HEART RATE MONITORING: Generally speaking, students who come to my classes have difficulty achieving the levels of intensity that are required for them to get the results they long for. The reason being that they may never have been involved in any competitive sports, they may have been a couch potato for the past twenty years. They are simply not used to seeking a level of mild discomfort in their exertions. There are, however, some serious exceptions to this and these people may have doctors' orders to keep their heart rate at a certain level and no higher. This is another important reason to have a dialogue with the instructor you have chosen, as they will generally expect that you want to be pushed to work harder. I am a big fan of what is termed **'THE TALK TEST'** or **'RATE OF**

PERCEIVED EXERTION (RPE): for water exercise as it is most difficult to stop moving and find a vein or artery to count pulses in the water... counter productive for most participants. Instead, I will suggest during various aerobic combinations or interval trainings, that we push for a seven, eight, or even nine on a scale of one to ten. Studies show that your perceived level of activity is usually quite accurate. As for the 'Talk Test', if you can say three words such as "I feel great!", then you generally are. If getting those three words out is a teensy bit difficult due to labored breathing then "Congratulations!", you are working with some real intensity. If you are a motor mouth, don't fool yourself about having a good cardiovascular workout, because you won't! (You may be enjoying many other valuable benefits of water exercise while chatting, but not the benefits of aerobic conditioning.) If you are uncertain or you fall into a high risk category, a waterproof heart rate monitor may be ideal for your needs (www.heartratewatchcompany.com). The easy **FORMULA** for determining your ideal exercise heart rate is: 220 minus your age = maximum heart rate you should achieve while exercising. Keep in mind that your heart rate will likely be up to seventeen beats per minute slower than that same level of exertion would read on land due to the unique properties of water.

SMOOTH MOVES AND SETS TO SPLASH DANCE

INTERVAL DRILLS: This is the easiest method to employ for maximizing aerobic benefits. It seems I read more good things about interval training all the time. A Canadian study showed that pushing toward your maximum heart rate (that eight or nine **RPE** for most people) will cause you to burn as many as four times your normal calories and also increase your caloric expenditure for the remainder of the day. The following is a simple set that's both fun and effective. You can use it repeatedly and vary the timing if you are a beginner training solo or if you want to incorporate intensity without struggling to remember lots of new steps. See Illustrations for **DRILLS** and **COMBINATION SETS** -

MAKING WAVES: SPLASH DANCE INTERVAL DRILLS

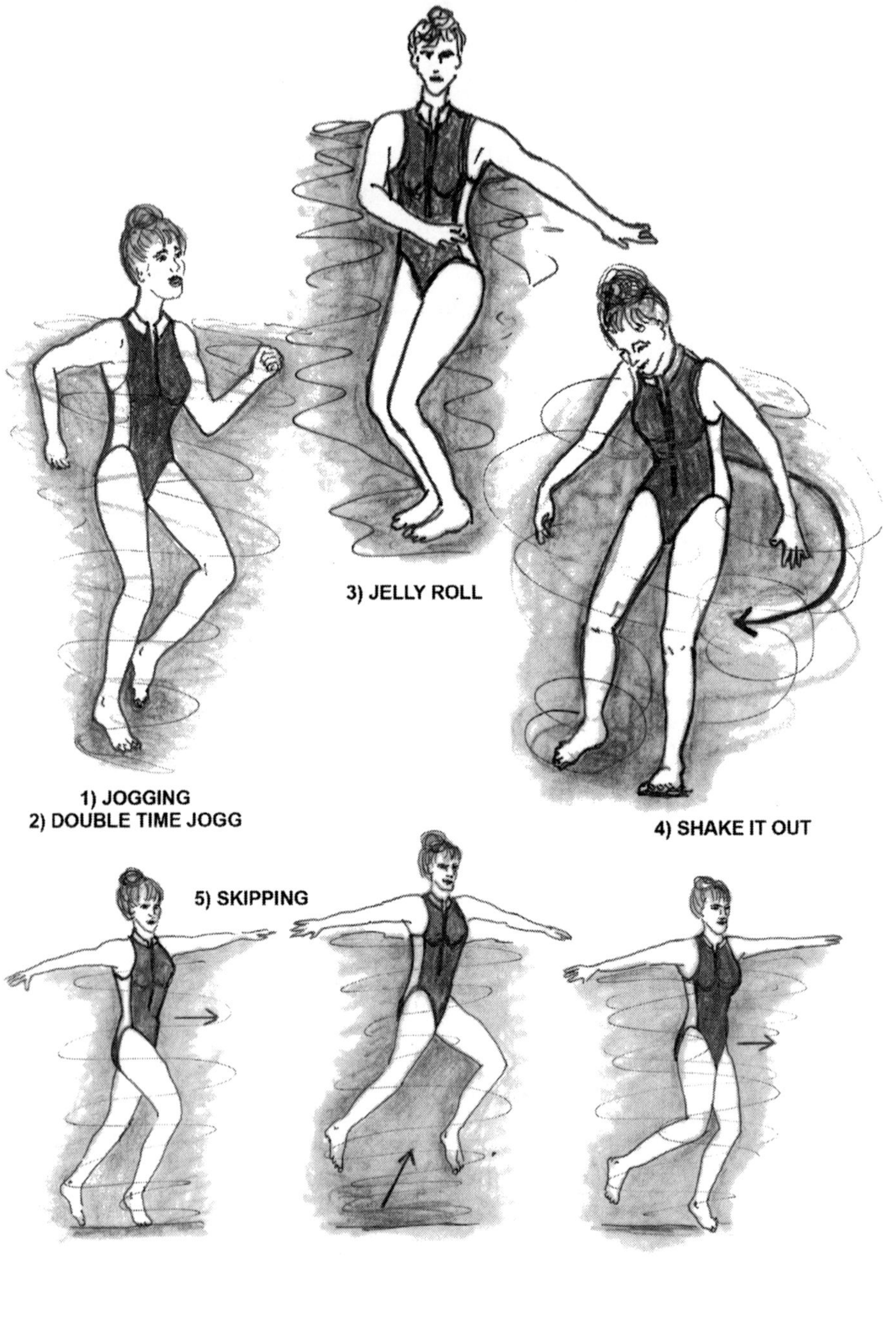

MAKING WAVES: SPLASH DANCE INTERVAL DRILLS CONTINUED

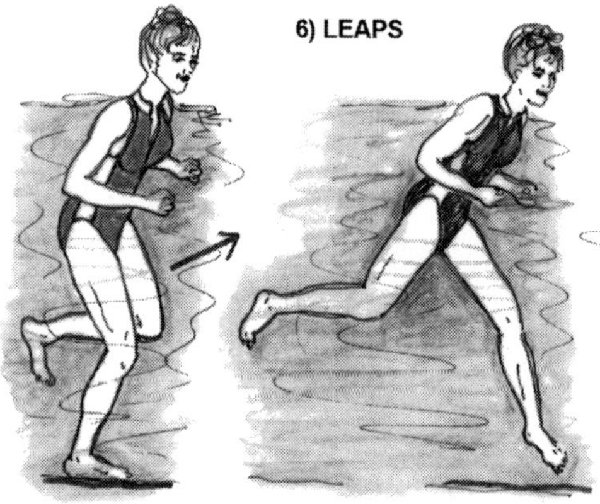

6) LEAPS

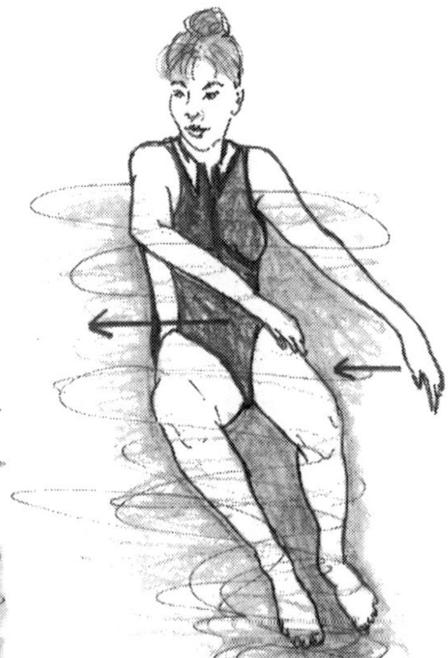

7) MOGUL TUCKS

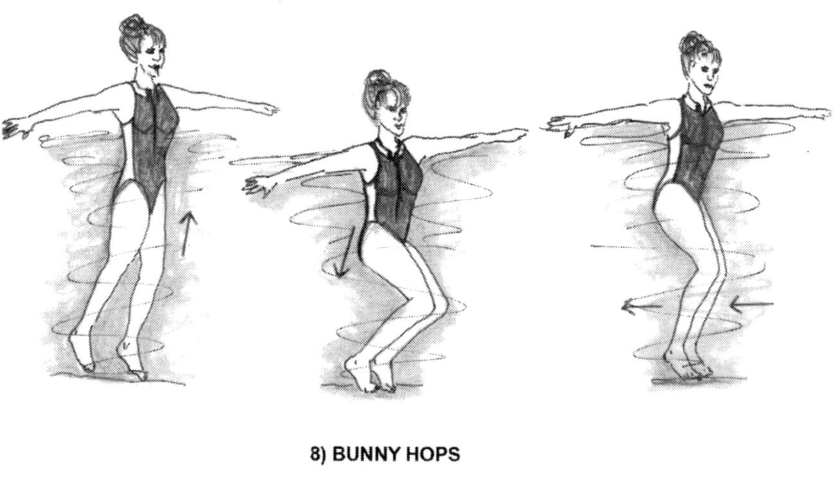

8) BUNNY HOPS

1) JOGGING: begin in chest high water, feet shoulder width apart, chest lifted, shoulders down, neck as relaxed as possible...focus on a really big range of motion (lifting the knees up high, while tucking the belly button up into the ribs, hands completely relaxed as you reach the opposite arm out over the knee that's coming up) - Begin to focus on your breathing, in through the nose out through the mouth... you can vary the timing on these intervals but thirty seconds is good for most beginners-

2) DOUBLE TIME JOG: now, let's step up the game with an interval, you will notice that your range of motion may get slightly shorter, keep your hands completely relaxed (they carry so much tension with digital devices, driving, etc. and the water massage will feel great) maintain your form and your breathing as above-

3) JELLY ROLL: Are you up for an intense interval now? Think of a belly dancer jogging or what is so unglamorously referred to as a 'jelly roll', your core muscles will be fully engaged, the hands are still relaxed- if you are very strong, you can take the movement into a circle and then reverse the circle... (In some yoga circles, the 'soft' tummy is embraced, so don't let a little jiggle here depress you!)

4) 'SHAKE IT OUT' afterward with a relaxing figure eight sway or circle where you stay down as much as possible (try to get some shoulder into the water by bending the knees a little more) and really let your arms go limp, if you move in a little circle, let the water pull your arms away from you... *I like to follow most of my intensity combinations with a variation of this relaxation technique* as it helps move lactic acid build up in the muscles- you will feel better later!

5) SKIPPING: coming to drills of greater effort now, beginning with an easy skip across the pool- seniors who haven't been able to skip on land in awhile will have a look of glee!

6) LEAPS across the pool are a vigorous way to please the cross trainers-lead with the right leg, then lead with the left leg- it's fun to try different hand positions...palms at the side slicing verses a cupped palm assist-

7) MOGUL TUCKS are very popular among skiers as it will strengthen the muscles they use on the slops while strengthening core and working balance. I like to pretend I have ski poles- reach out with long arms and dig (cup you palm and pull water towards you) down to the right as you vigorously propel the body right. Next follow to the left, and alternate across the pool-

8) BUNNY HOPS are very similar but the emphasis is on hopping forward without a strong arm assist, core challenge and balance are emphasized-**HIPPITY HOP** backwards is fun too!

COMBINATION SETS: I am going to give you some of my favorites here but don't be afraid to develop your own, particularly if you have natural dance ability. One thing I might mention now is the use of **'LONG LEVERS'** versus **'SHORT LEVERS'** in your water workout. If you make a movement with a long arm or a long leg, we call it using a long lever. While using a long lever may be much more challenging to the core, many participants in a class have issues (bad backs, hip and/ or knee replacements, etc.) that make a short lever variation (bending of the knee or elbow) of a step more appropriate in the interest of having the workout without causing further pain or risking injury. With most of the following moves, I like to use dumbbells, and there are various sizes to choose from as well as movements that can be performed with the dumbbell under the shoulders when some support is helpful. Additionally, there are participants who need to forego dumbbells and use the hands in assisting or impeding the movement. Try variations such as leading with the wide surface of the palm versus a slicing action of the palm turned sideways. Not to get too complicated...do what feels good! If something hurts you, don't do it. I tell new participants in class not to worry about getting it right for awhile, it's better to enjoy what you are able to do, get the benefits, and come back regularly. *Consistency* is key to progress in exercise!

1) CROSS COUNTRY SKING: has been a traditional staple of water exercise and it's easy to understand why. It's the variations I do that make it fun... try adding a little **bounce**, a **PLYOMETRIC** (propelled) variation is great for the fitter participant... really push off the bottom of the pool and land with the opposite ski in front... try a **suspended** variation without touching the bottom of the pool, punching the opposite dumbbell out over the leg in front (here we could put the dumbbells under the shoulders for support)... think of jumping hurdles without touching ground and try to kick your buttocks with the heel in back (good luck with that!)- here you really feel that you are carving out the core muscles of the trunk, very intense without going fast... use your exhale to power through the movements...

MAKING WAVES: SPLASH DANCE COMBINATION SETS

1) CROSS COUNTRY SKI
VARIATIONS:
with DUMBBELLS
with a BOUNCE
with a TUCK
PROPELLED
SUSPENDED

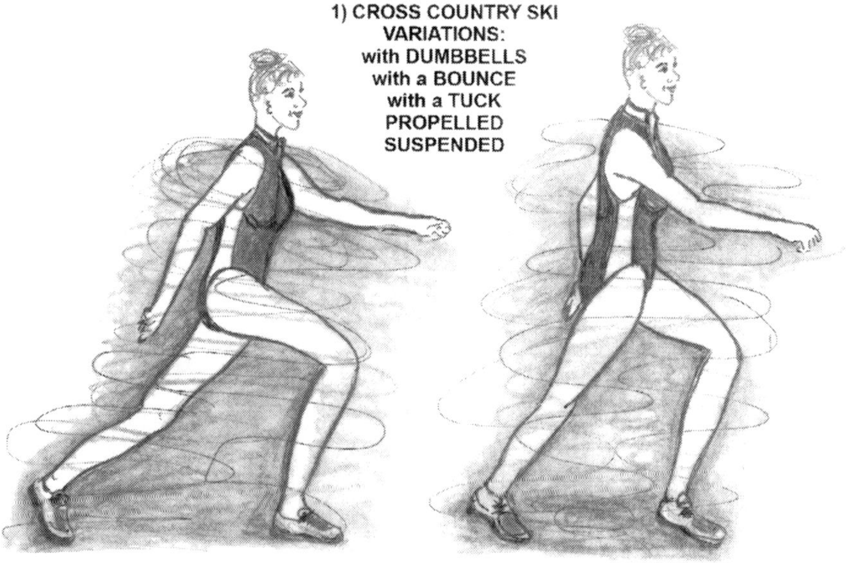

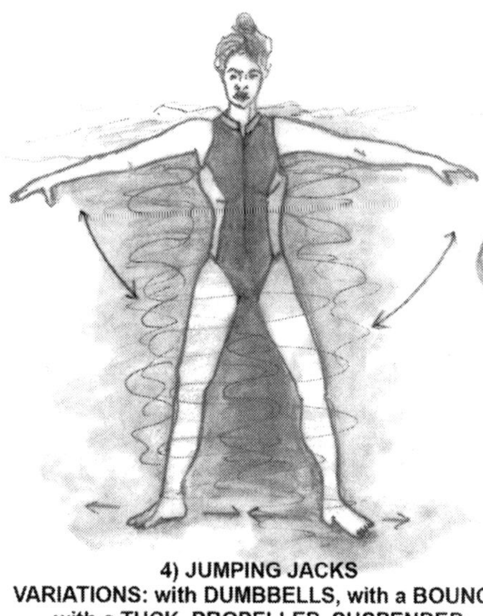

4) JUMPING JACKS
VARIATIONS: with DUMBBELLS, with a BOUNCE
with a TUCK, PROPELLED, SUSPENDED
5) SINGLE LEG KICK with a JACK
6) CROSSOVER JACKS

2) LUNGING
SITE TO SIDE
with a PUNCH

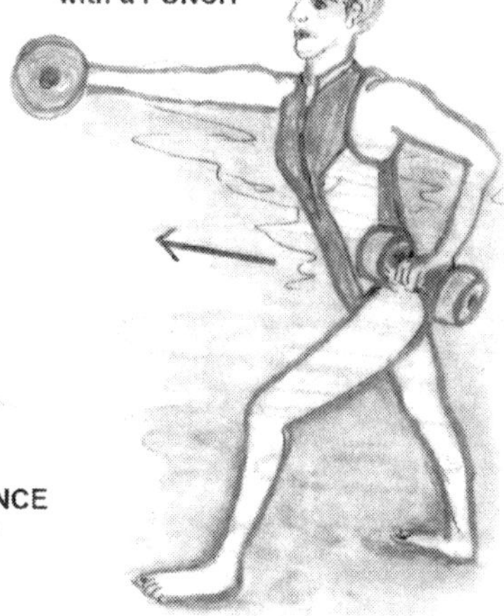

MAKING WAVES: SPLASH DANCE COMBINATION SETS CONTINUED

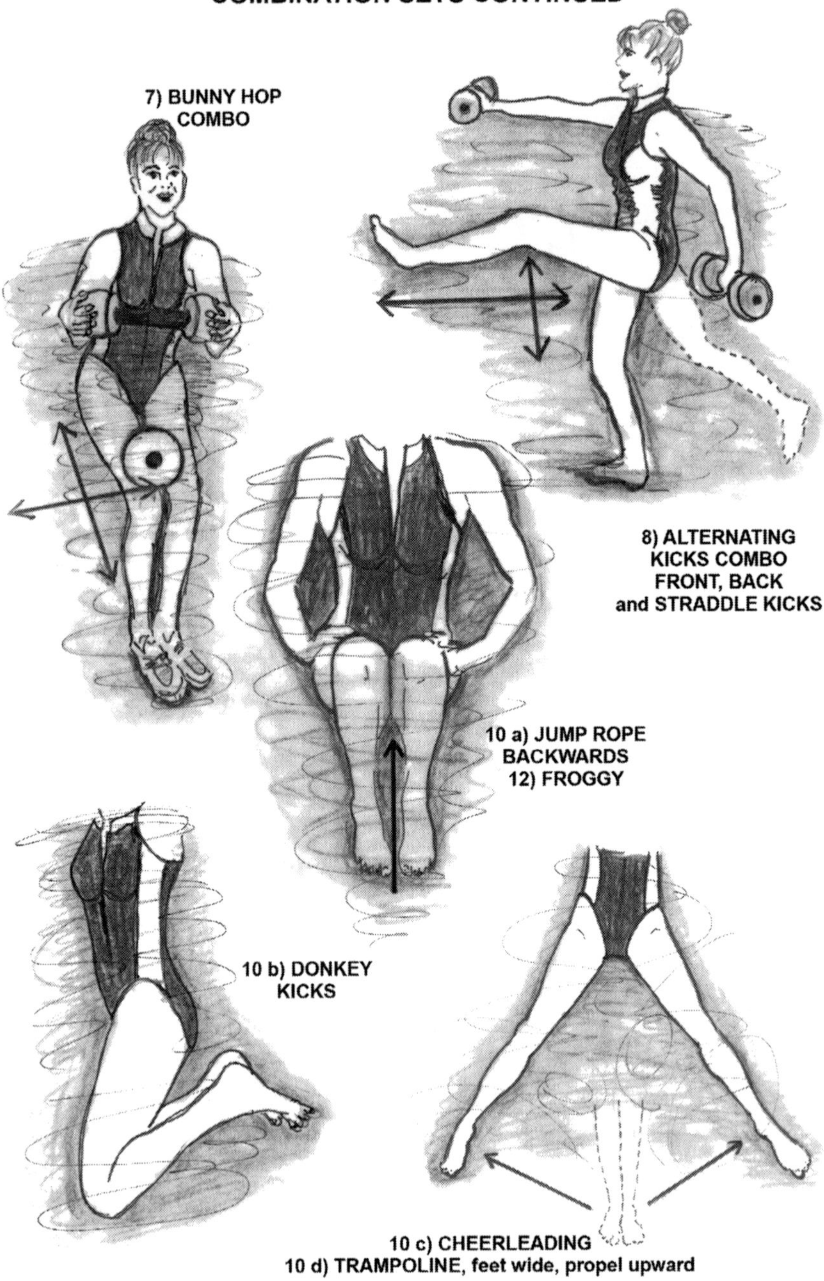

2) LUNGING SIDE to SIDE: can be a very effective transition from the cross country style lunge (above)- try focusing on the stretch, going further with the lunge than you would on land as the water supports you and massages your muscles, next try bumping up the intensity with some kickboxing inspiration- add a bounce and a **PUNCH!**

3) SEMI CIRCLE HOPS: now pull the feet together, and keep the elbows bent- 180 degree semi-circle hops, side to side (feet, hips and shoulders move together)... feel how you're leading with your hips here- for fun, try the dumbbells overhead and lead with the momentum of your arms, then back to the surface of the water with the dumbbells and lead with the hips again-

4) JUMPING JACKS: next bring the feet wider apart transitioning to a jumping jack, try pushing the dumbbells down as you bring your feet together for added buoyancy (only if you can keep your shoulders down)-try adding variations like little **bounces** to the jack... in with a bounce and out with a bounce... try another propelled **PLYOMETRIC** version by pushing off the bottom of the pool keeping the knees slightly bent and trying to kick your buttocks with your heels-

5) SINGLE LEG KICK with a JACK: next, it's an easy transition to try pushing the dumbbell down with the supporting leg that stays down, the hips are facing forward and the knee (of the leg you're kicking up) faces the surface of the water-

6) CROSSOVER JACKS: crossing the midline of the body alternating arm and leg on top in this intense version of a **JACK** (you might be better off attempting this initially without the dumbbells; try cupping the palms of your hands), keeping the elbows slightly bent... for the very strong, a **SUSPENDED** variation is great fun but do try and keep your neck as relaxed as possible - (hip replacement recipients should never cross the midline, but you knew that!)

7) BUNNY HOP COMBO: shake it out, as described in the previous section, then take one dumbbell and place the handle between your thighs (keeping the feet and knees together), then lightly clasp the ends of the remaining dumbbell with your hands... reaching the hands out in front first (dumbbell on the surface of the water), **jump forward,** with the feet and then **backward** - next extend the hand held dumbbell to the side and then hop to that side, then back to center... it should feel as though you're pulling the feet **forward and back, side and center**- repeat -8x-, change sides for -8x-, then make it even more of a core challenge by **TRAVELING** with it (**alternating sides** creates more resistance from the water), -8x- or more-

8) ALTERNATING KICKS COMBO: front, back, and side to side, straddle kicks, taking the dumbbells back into the hands, go for:

a) ALTERNATING KICKS in FRONT: punching the opposite dumbbell out over the leg going up, - 8x- followed by:

b) ALTERNATING KICKS to the REAR: dumbbells together, arms going side to side in opposition to the leg (you might want to pass on this if your back has been bothering you), -8x- followed by:

c) ALTERNATING SIDE to SIDE STRADDLE KICKS: motion of the dumbbell going down with the leg going down - 8x- after 4 rounds of this (front, back and sides) - I like to *break* this set up with:

d) ALTERNATING TOE TOUCH: (feet wide apart, opposite dumbbell to the toe in front, try to keep a little bounce going when you return to the wide leg position), - 8x- followed by:

e) ALTERNATING HEEL TOUCH: (opposite dumbbell to the heel in back), - 8x- then:

f) ALTERNATING STRADDLE KICKS repeated - 8x- then:

g) REPEAT the entire alternating kicks combo (**a,b,c,**) in sets of - 4x- adding a **QUARTER TURN** after each set, make a complete circle (4 sets) and then **REVERSE** the circle, next go for the **toe touch, heel touch combo again** - finish with one more round (**a,b,c,**) of - 2x- kicks, **REVERSE again**- Wow, you are one tough cookie! Check your heart rate?

9) UP, OVER, DOWN IN FRONT: (not for those with joint issues!) resting the hands on the dumbbell with the elbows soft, reach the long arms all the way out in front, then make a big circle to the rear, **work your full range of motion** with one bent knee under your chin, other long leg straight out in back, after enjoying the water massage momentarily (note that dumbbells can go under the shoulders for support), start to focus on your **ABDOMINALS** as you bring the long arms forward- tuck that belly button up into the ribs, next- bump it up to **long arms going down in front** as you lift your knees up into the chest, extending the long legs slowly out in front and then down to pool bottom... I like to save the **REVERSE** (long arms going down in back) until after I've done another high intensity combination-

10) JUMP ROPE BACKWARDS - COMBO: imagine the jumprope in your hands (cupping your palms to create resistance) taking it under the heels in back, focus on lifting the knees as this is the recovery portion of this intense combination set - 8x-, followed by an explosive-

a) PUSH: off the bottom of the pool, reaching long arms up - 8x-, then back to jumping rope - 8x -, repeat the push - 8x-, followed by:

b) DONKEY KICKS: (kicking the heels to the buttocks and reaching the long arms up - 8x-, going back to toe touch, knee lift -8x-, repeat the jumps - 8x-, then the donkey kicks - 8x-, then add:

c) CHEERLEADING KICKS: (feet together then push off the bottom kicking legs out to the sides) - 8x-, go back to toe touch, knee lift - 8x-, repeat the jumps, donkey kicks, cheerleading kicks, and adding:

d) TRAMPOLINE KICKS: (feet wider, pushing off the bottom - -8x-... for more fun with intensity, go for sets of - 4x -, followed by - 2x -, (the recovery toe touch knee lift combo can be longer) **NOTE:** this is a good time to do a talk test or RPE to see if you are working at your optimal potential-

11) RECOVERY SET: moving with a large **STEP TAP**, **STEP KICK** to the **right**, followed by step tap, step kick to the **left**, repeat - 2x-, then, step tap step kick **forwards**, followed by step tap, step kick **backwards**, repeat- 2x-, then take it to the sides again, forward and back as desirable allowing the arms to relax and be pulled away from the body or using arms to assist a more vigorous movement-

12) FROGGY: with feet shoulder width apart, and knee's bent, begin with a light **toe touch, knee lift** while **treading water** with the **hands**-8x-, then push vigorously off the bottom of the pool while also pushing the flat palms of the hands from the waters surface to the thighs, repeat -8x-, and then increase intensity by bringing the flat palms of the hands together and pressing them down between the thighs -8x-, followed by still more intensity as you kick the heels up towards the buttocks and reach the long arms up overhead -8x-, then repeat from the top in sets of 4-

13) THE TWIST: with feet and arms (hands relaxed) wide apart and a good bend in the knees, begin to work this old 60's dance step (make sure the back feels good!) then you can pick up the intensity by adding cupped palms - 8x-, followed by trying to kick the opposite cheek of your buttocks with the heel in back - 8x-, then adding arms overhead - 8x-, follow with sets of 4 and quarter turns-

14) THE CAN CAN: a very friendly group 'can-can' have a lotta fun with this, especially if you include an authentic musical selection. It helps to place your arm across your neighbor's shoulder as water provides a lot more resistance than the skirts of yore- In a line dance formation, lift the knee, tap the toe to the floor, then kick the long leg up- if you're a strong group, move it across the pool, and then reverse legs as well as direction- Shorter sets will offer up more challenge with increased resistance from the water-

15) TAKE A FREE RIDE! In a splashy take on traditional folk dancing, have your group (they must be in reasonably strong condition!) form a big circle, hold hands and expand the size of the circle as much as possible while they start to pick up speed heading in one direction (it helps to have them face that direction as opposed to the center which they might normally do on land). Having chosen the candidate for a free ride (birthday anyone?), wait until everyone is moving forcefully and then let the rider lift their long legs out in front and squeal in glee! This is great fun but I've had to abandon it on occasion when my group turns out to be unable to move forcefully with speed :(

16) DO IT YOURSELF - create your own combination: try knee lifts or jazz kicks followed by heel jacks, add a plyometric jump, kick the heels up in back, add a turn, then repeat... whatever floats your boat! If you're good at this, and you like working with people, consider taking a certification training- (www.aea.com) with baby boomers retiring in droves, there will be more demand for good instructors. Another recent development in aquatic equipment is the treadmill and bike available from www. hydrorider.com. While these can be great for the solo exerciser, there's a cycling class I'd like to teach!

MAKING WAVES: 'CHILL' NOW

"I pray to be like the ocean, with soft currents,
maybe waves at times.
More and more, I want the consistency
rather than the highs and the lows."
~ Drew Barrymore

"A person has three choices in life.
You can swim against the tide and get
exhausted, or you can tread water
and let the tide sweep you away, or you can
swim with the tide and let it take you
where it wants you to go."
~ Diane Frolov & Andrew Schneider

"Sit in reverie and watch the changing color
of the waves that break upon the idle
seashore of the mind."
~ Henry Wadsworth Longfellow

COOLING DOWN: STRETCH AND RELAX

Feel free to go back to **A Thermal Warm-up,** which I presented at the beginning of **MAKING WAVES**. Take at least 5 minutes to cross the pool in some of the various ways, which

I described there. Your emphasis should now be on letting go of any muscular tension that you may have acquired during the aerobic portion of class. Pay special attention to allowing the hands (no dumbbells!), shoulders and neck to remain relaxed. Stay submerged as much as possible so the water can massage your chest and back as you move forward and backwards. You can finish up with the **Big Circle** or **Figure Eight,** which were described under **A More Focused Stretch**. When you're ready for more, there is a whole new world for you to explore by bringing what you may have already studied from Yoga, Tai Chi, and Pilates to the water. I'm going to offer you two different approaches to ending your water workout now, see illustrations –

STANDING YOGA POSES: after crossing the pool as above, come to a stationary position in chest high water with the feet shoulder width apart, **knees** slightly **bent** (note that this is key to balance throughout the poses), and do **The Figure Eight,** progressing to **Infinity** if your back is strong, as it will really carve out your abdominals as you swing your long arms and cupped palms up from one knee towards the opposite shoulder, flexing the abs on the downswing (from the shoulder down towards the knee and back up to the opposite shoulder)- After a few repetitions, try taking both **long arms** around in **back**, **clasping** the **hands** together and **pressing up**, then **releasing** your hands...

1) POINT and FLEX POSE: bringing the feet closer together and keeping your left knee slightly bent, clasp your **hands** around the right calf as you **lift the right leg up** perpendicular to the body- **point your toes, flex your heel, circle your ankle,** and **reverse** the circle –

MAKING WAVES: 'CHILL' NOW STANDING YOGA POSES

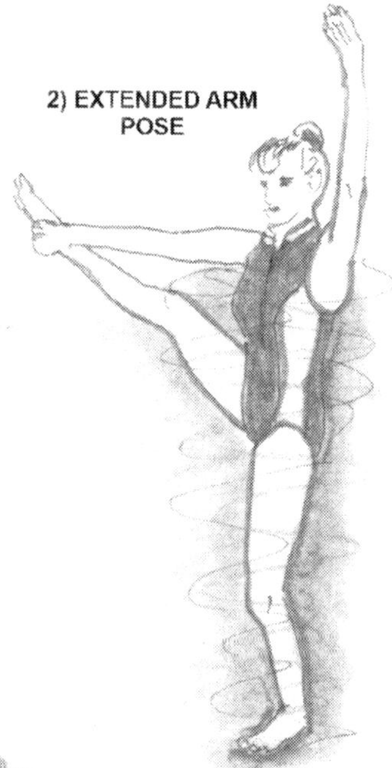

2) EXTENDED ARM POSE

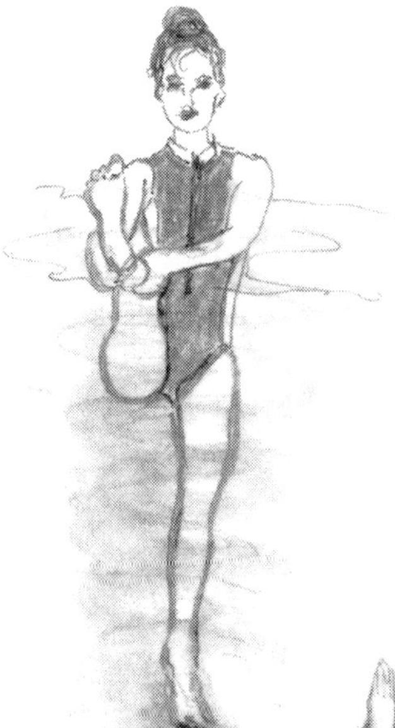

1) POINT and FLEX POSE

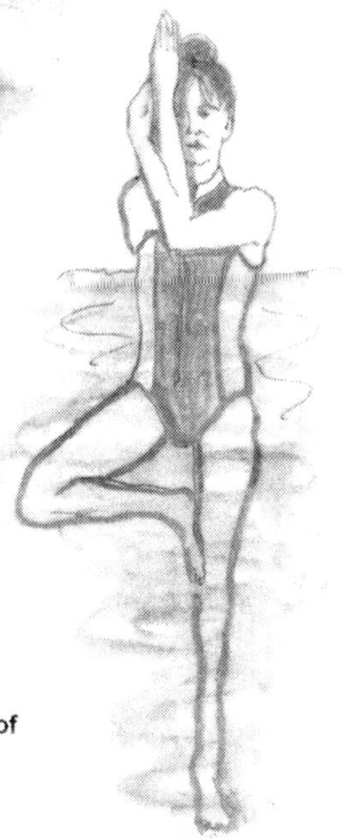

3) POSE of a TREE

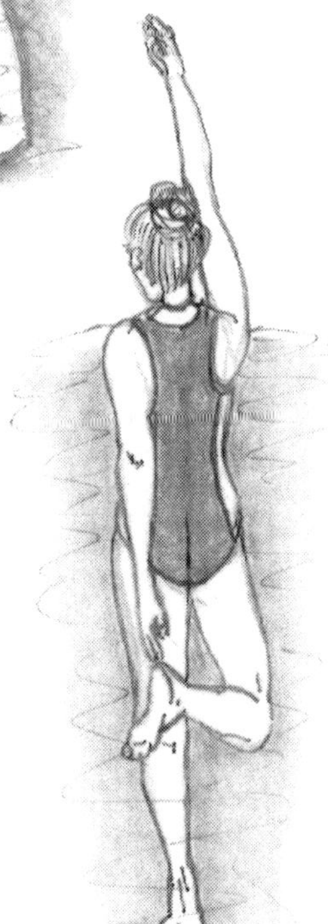

4) RUNNERS POSE

MAKING WAVES: 'CHILL' NOW STANDING YOGA POSES CONTINUED

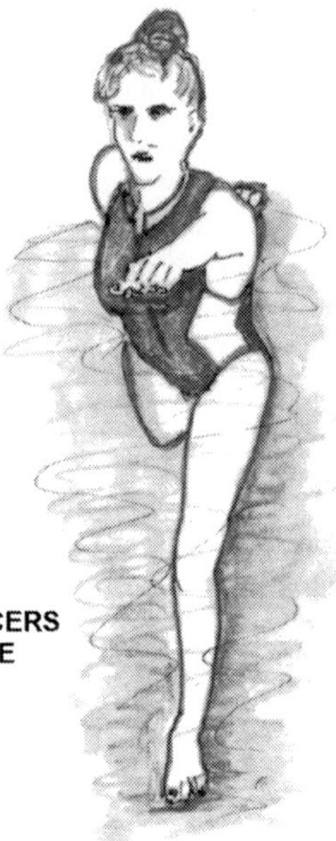

5) DANCERS POSE

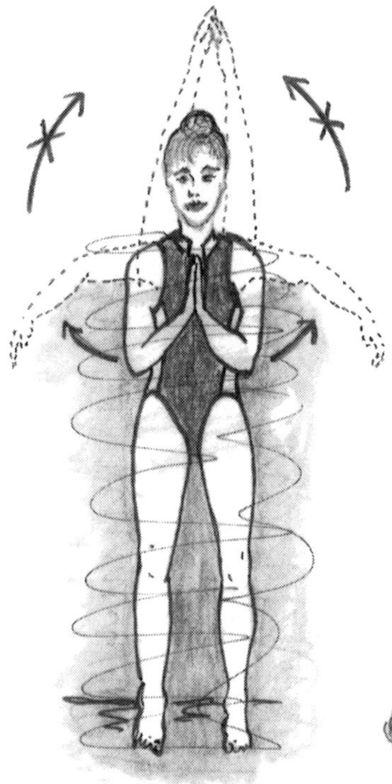

7) REVERSE LEG NUMBERS 1-6
8) MOUNTAIN POSE

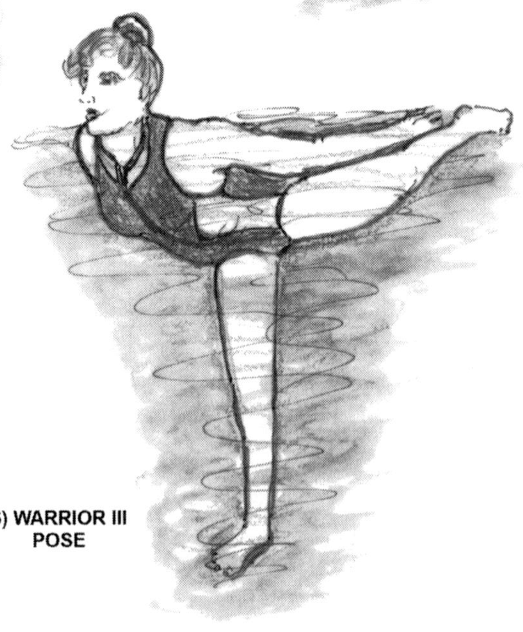

6) WARRIOR III POSE

2) EXTENDED ARM POSE: next take the right arm around the outside of the right knee and lock it underneath the leg, **opening** it towards your right and reaching overhead with the left arm as you pause to work your balance, if you are very flexible, you can reach over your knee and cup your right hand over the heel of the foot - then **extend** the **right leg** and **arm up** and **out** to the right, holding this pose and breathing deeply as you experience the ease of working your **balance** in water-

3) POSE of a TREE: In a smooth transition, bring the **right foot** to the **inner thigh** of the left leg and lock it there as you reach both long arms overhead, balance and breathe deeply- (the fitter participant can get more complicated: cross the right arm over the left at the elbow, then cross again at the wrist bringing the palms together), inhaling and reaching up as far as possible then exhaling as you return to the chest-

4) RUNNER'S POSE: Next clasp the foot again and swing it around behind you, rotating the hip as you bring the **knees** close together, and the **heel** up towards the **buttocks**- raise your **left arm** straight up, balancing and breathing into the stretch-

5) DANCER'S POSE: Now bending forward at the **waist**, and continuing to reach the **left arm** out (parallel to/or resting on the water, hips facing forward and down) – inhale deeply in this position, shoot that oxygen down the spine, and feel it lengthen as you breath -repeat the breathing, be kind to your spine...

6) WARRIOR III POSE: Releasing the **arms**, reach them both out in front as you now extend that **right foot** fully behind you, pushing away with the pointed toe in this pose. I like to swing **both arms** around parallel to the leg as it is so easy and exhilarating to work your balance in the water-

7) REVERSE the SERIES: drop the leg and breath deeply as you reach both arms overhead, coming back to the standing position and then begin again -now keeping the **right knee** slightly bent (again, key to your balance) and lifting the long **left leg** up in front-

8) MOUNTAIN POSE: finally, keeping the feet shoulder width apart, inhale deeply reaching both long **arms overhead** and **clasping thumbs**- press the arms to the **right** slightly, to the **left**, and then **release** the hands and inhaling deeply, reach out to the **sides** and **straight up** once more... I like to finish this series by bringing my fingertips to the back of the neck, rubbing out any muscle tension that may have accumulated there and then pressing the elbows back with a last focused exhale-

SIDE OF THE POOL COOL DOWN: This is an alternative combination that I do when my class is small and there will be sufficient room along the sides of the pool as well as corners and stairs if you care to focus on the abdominals as well... Begin the cool down by **crossing the pool** as described, continuing with the **figure eight** and then:

MAKING WAVES: 'CHILL' NOW
SIDE OF THE POOL COOL DOWN

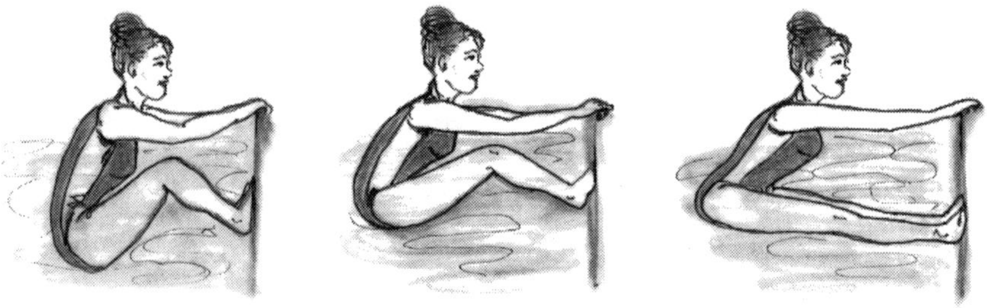

5) CLIMB THE WALL

6) LUNGE
swing to the right
swing to the left

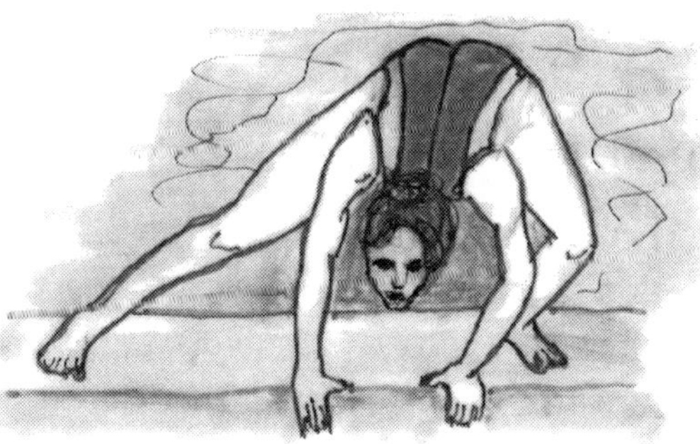

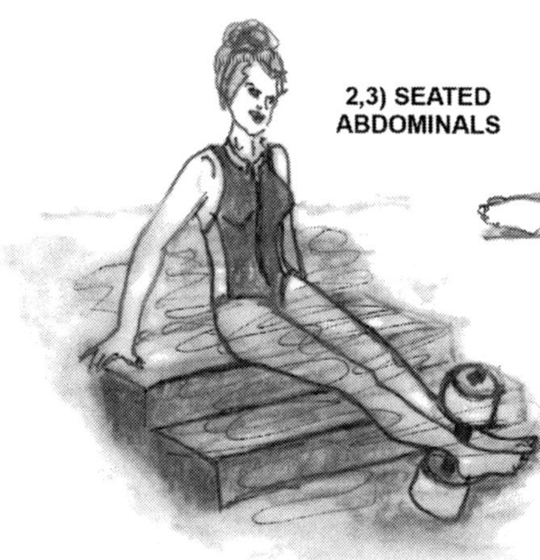

2,3) SEATED
ABDOMINALS

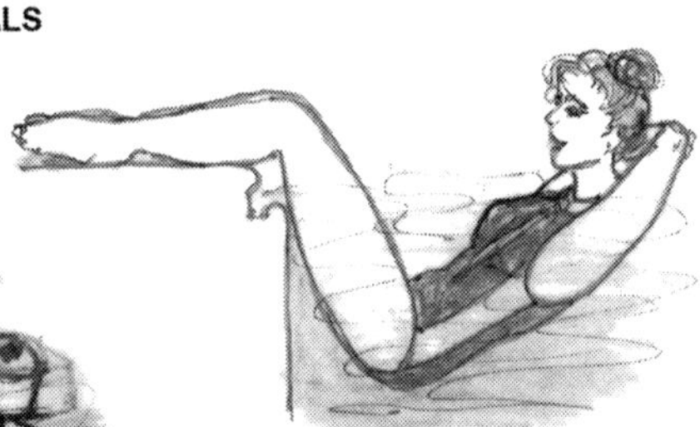

7) HANGING
ABDOMINALS

1) ABDOMINALS: coming to the stairs (you can do this seated on stairs if there is a railing to hold) or corner of your pool, support your upper body by clasping the sides of the pool (from the corners)- now lift the long legs straight up in front, then bending the knees, **pull both knees in towards the right armpit**, extend the legs straight out again, then bending the knees, **pull both knees in towards the left armpit**- If it feels good, add more intensity, really turning your torso into the movement, focusing on the exhale as you contract the abs-

2) ABDOMINALS with RESISTANCE: in this same start position, lift the legs and **bending the right knee, cross it over the thigh** of the long left leg... now **bend the left leg** pulling it into your torso with this added resistance- after several repetitions, **reverse the legs** and repeat-

3) ABDOMINALS with a DUMBBELL: in the same start position, **add a dumbbell,** squeezing the handle **between the thighs** - now try to push your legs down and then control the upward motion- repeat as desired but do not attempt this if your back is less than terrific-

4) ACHILLES TENDON, calf muscle stretch: coming to the sides of the pool now, in chest high water, begin by facing the wall and resting the hands on it, bring the right toes to the wall with the right knee bent and the long left leg extended straight behind you - **push down** firmly but gently into the back left heel, breathing deeply - then **reverse** legs-

5) CLIMB the WALL: with a good hand grip on the wall, begin to **climb** up it with the knees bent- when the knees reach the torso, contract your abdominals and gently push your hips away from the wall, straightening the legs- if this feels very good, bend the knees again and climb up another inch or so and **repeat**-

6) LUNGE: against the wall by swinging the bent right knee more to the right and lengthening the left leg against the wall and then **reversing** the leg-

7) ADVANCED ABDOMINALS: for the very fit or for those who can enlist a 'spotter' to hold your ankles over the side of the pool, support your head gently with both arms keeping the elbows open, taking care not to pull on the neck and descend into the water as far as is comfortable for you...

8) TURNING AWAY FROM THE WALL: with the heels against it and the arms behind you, hands securely holding the wall, start to pull your torso away from the wall- drop your chin, roll the right ear towards the right shoulder and then repeat with the left side-

9) FINISH: by walking away from the wall, bend the knees, arms down, and then slowly straighten the knees as you inhale and reach both long arms up overhead (locking thumbs if it feels good), exhaling and pressing the arms to the right, inhale- reaching up again, then exhale and press arms to the left, reach straight up again, and then come down to the bent knee position one last time, inhaling, reaching straight up, and focus on lengthening the spine with a slow exhale...

MAKING WAVES: 'CHILL' NOW
SIDE OF THE POOL BALLET BARRE INSPIRED

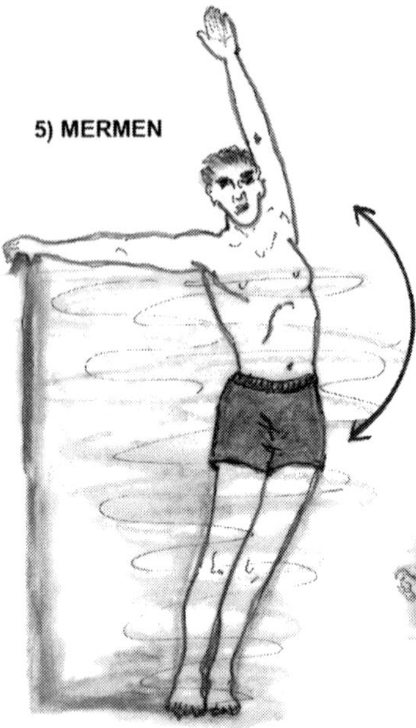

5) MERMEN

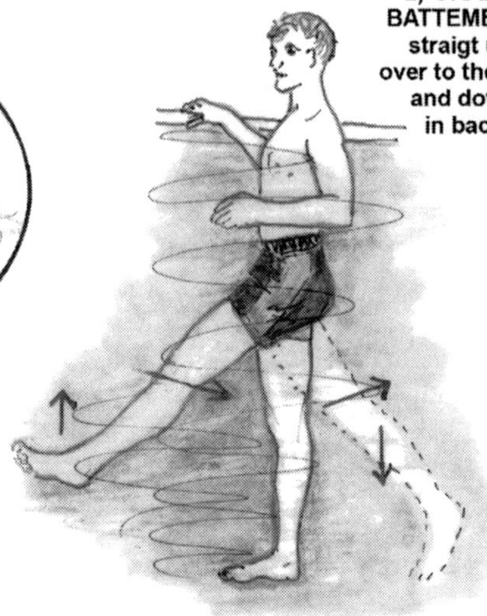

2) GRAND BATTEMENTS
straigt up
over to the side
and down
in back

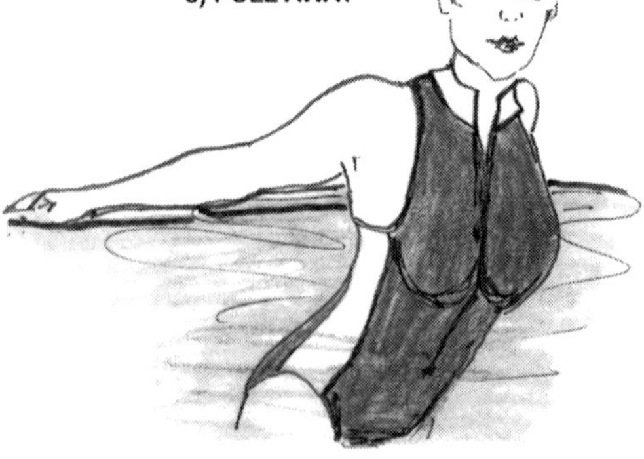

8) PULL AWAY

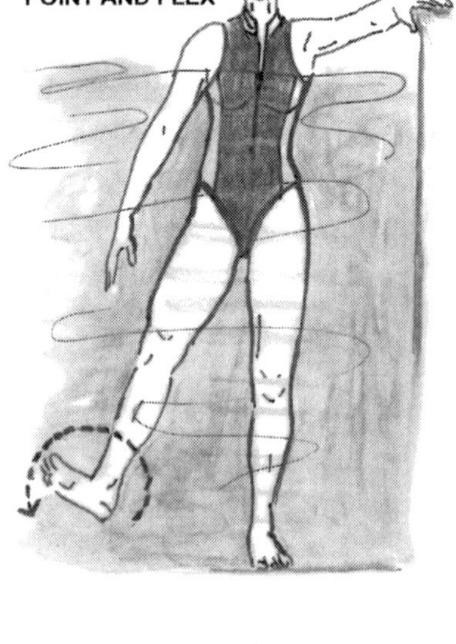

4) DEGAGE
FRONT PLUS
POINT AND FLEX

SIDE OF THE POOL BALLET BARRE INSPIRED EXERCISES: The following are an alternative and fun way to finish a shallow water session. The aquajogger leg cuff really puts them over the top for the fitter participant as the upward motion must be controlled due to increased buoyancy and the downward motions encounter more resistance-

1) ACHILLES TENDON, calf muscle stretch: as described in the previous section **#4)** again facing the pool wall-

2) GRAND BATTEMENTS: turning your right side to the wall now and gently gripping it with your fingertips, keep your chest lifted and shoulders down as you lift that outside left leg **straight up** in **front**, pointing the toes, swing it over to the **side** , and then straight **back,** and **down**. It's important to maintain a neutral spine here (pull that belly button up into the ribs!) so keep the torso lifted, and don't go beyond the range of motion where you are in control of the torso.

3) BATTEMENT TENDU: next, bring that long leg straight up at the **side**, pointing the toes, and then digging down through the heel and crossing in **front** of the standing leg as you push towards the wall- then straight up at the side again, digging it down toward the wall **behind** the standing leg- repeat -8x-, or as desired-

4) DEGAGE FRONT PLUS: take that same left leg straight out in **front** about 10 inches from the bottom of the pool, toes pointed, and make a basketball sized **circle,** going as fast as you can (without moving your upright torso), then **reverse** the direction, digging down and back through the **heel-**

5) BARRE MERMAIDS (MERMEN?): with flat feet together, still gently clasping the side of the pool with the right hand, reach the long **left arm** all the way out towards the water leaning your body into it as well and then reaching up overhead. Note, this feels wonderful as long as you are able to comfortably grip the side of the pool...you can stretch much further than on land as you could only fall into water!

6) DEGAGE REAR: I like to face the pool wall, a relaxed arms length from the wall, gently clasping the wall, point the toes straight up in back, then dig the heel down. Focus on carving out the abdominals on that down swing- switch legs here, repeat, and then-

7) REVERSE SIDES REPEATING #'s 2, 3, 4, and 5: dedicated ballet lovers- add a **plié** routine to the above, my focus here is on what benefits from the addition of leg cuffs- In finishing up this series, **climb the wall** if you like, **lunging** as was explained in the **yoga** inspired moves, in **II - 5** above-

8) PULL AWAY: A favorite of mine is to face away from the wall with hands placed a little wider than the shoulders- firmly clasping the pool rim, enjoy pulling away, swinging toward the right and the left, releasing the shoulders, then drop the chin and work a little semi-circle with the neck-

MORE 'CHILL' - ICE IS NICE!: I find nearly universal negligence exists when it comes to icing injuries properly. (I understand because I, too, have been very guilty!) Like many people, it's easy to think "I'll work through this injury, it may not be so bad if I can keep moving... " When, in fact, you are setting yourself up for further tissue damage, increased inflammation, and more pain with this strategy (or, like me, simply negligence). You may recall the acronym **RICE,** a formula meant to be used immediately after hurting yourself. These simple steps can dramatically reduce the time it takes to heal and get back to your normal routine:

Rest- this is the simplest and most effective thing you can do. Unless the injury is severe, absolute rest should not exceed forty-eight hours because your muscles will start to stiffen-up and scar tissue around the injury will tighten-up. So, try and begin a little gentle exercise as soon as the initial pain and swelling subside-

Ice- apply immediately to injured area, either placing cubes in a plastic bag or choosing frozen vegetables such as peas for this purpose only as they will thaw and refreeze. Ice is a natural pain reliever and anti-inflammatory. It slows down blood flow to the area, reduces internal bleeding, and swelling while cutting your healing time in half. Wrap the ice in a soft towel and apply to the injured area for ten - twenty minutes before taking a break to prevent frostbite. Repeat as often as possible, at least once every hour when treating a new injury. For injuries that are healing well, even a short three minutes of ice after exercise will do much to drive away inflammation and insure continued speedy healing...

Compression- applying an elastic type tensor bandage to the area can help prevent swelling but be careful not to make it too tight as that might cut-off circulation-

Elevation- If the injured area is on an arm or leg, elevate the extremity above your heart level-

MAKING WAVES: USE YOUR NOODLE

"The higher your energy level,
the more efficient your body.
The more efficient your body,
the better you feel and the more you will use
your talent to produce outstanding results."
~ Anthony Robbins

"I never drink water because
of the disgusting things fish do in it."
~ W.C. Fields

This may be the only time you've read the statement 'use your noodle' when it's intended to be strictly literal. Sometimes called logs or Sqoodles, approximately 5 feet long...this kind of noodle can be oodles of fun! I've mentioned its use a couple times for support of injured people and in a variation of water walking. It can give more stability to those who are weak but it can also be used to take your workout to a more challenging level. Creating more challenge requires a more athletic noodle for most participants and I recommend the AquaJogger square sided Sqoodles, which are available at www.aquajogger.com. I frequently enjoy doing a half hour or more with my class using a noodle and I will share these exercises with you in a graduating level of difficulty. See illustrations -

MAKING WAVES: USE YOUR NOODLE
AEROBIC NOODLING

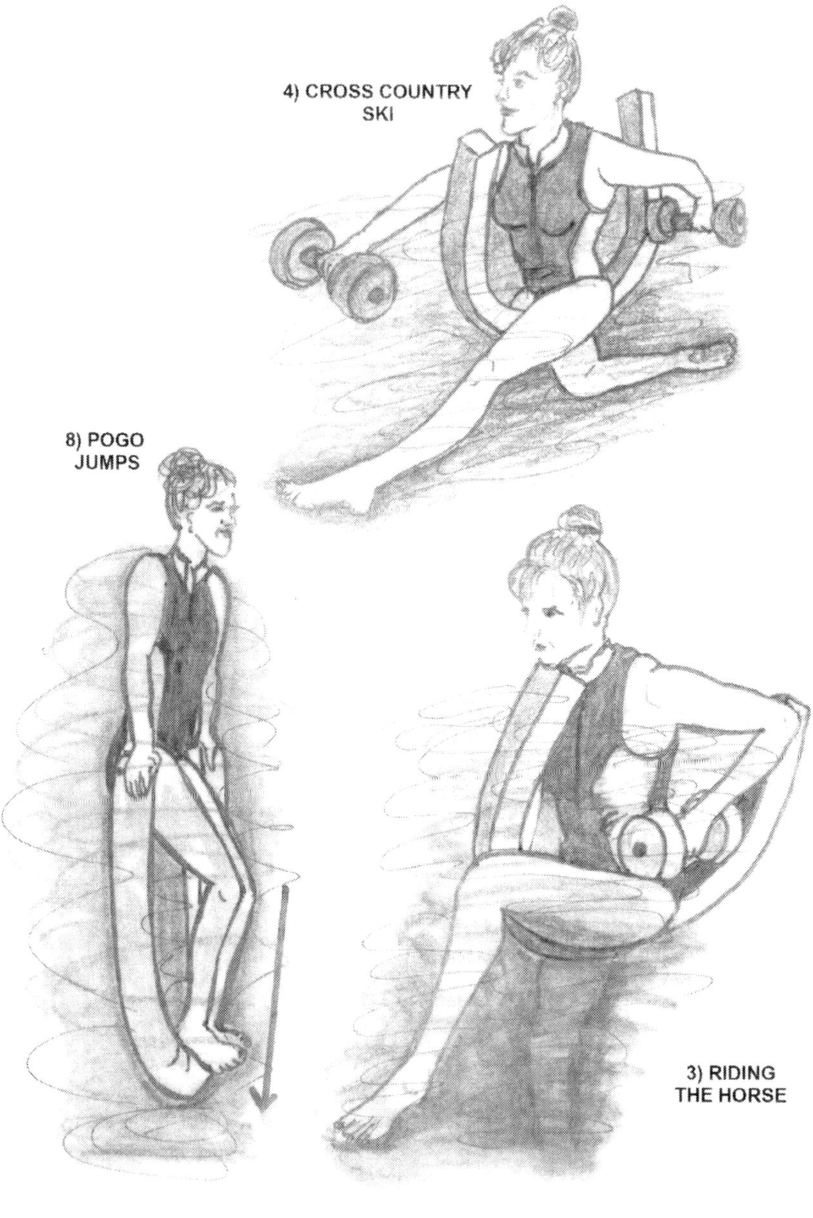

MAKING WAVES: USE YOUR NOODLE
AEROBIC NOODLING CONTINUED

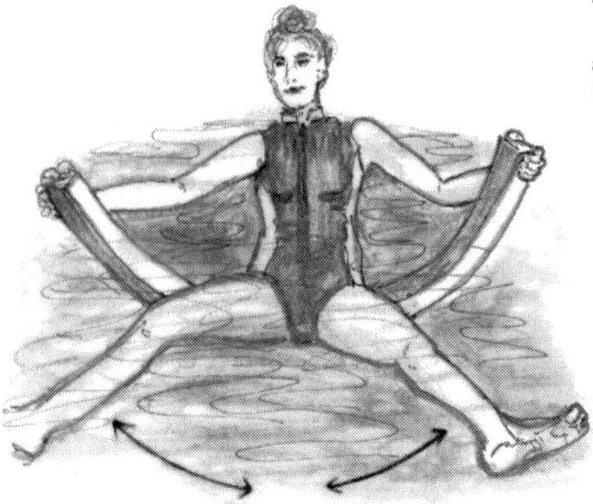

7) SITTING in a SWING
b) scissors open

7) SITTING in
a SWING
a) alternating
kicks in front

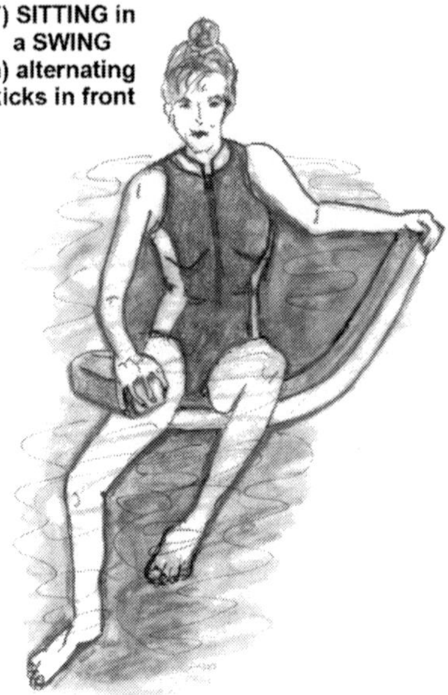

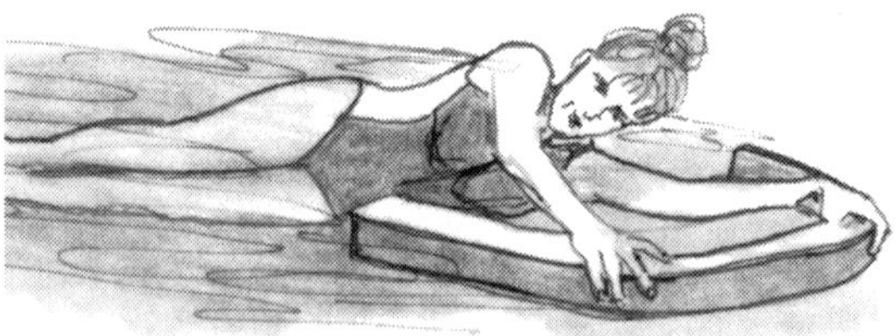

9) PUSH AWAYS
10) PUSH and PULL

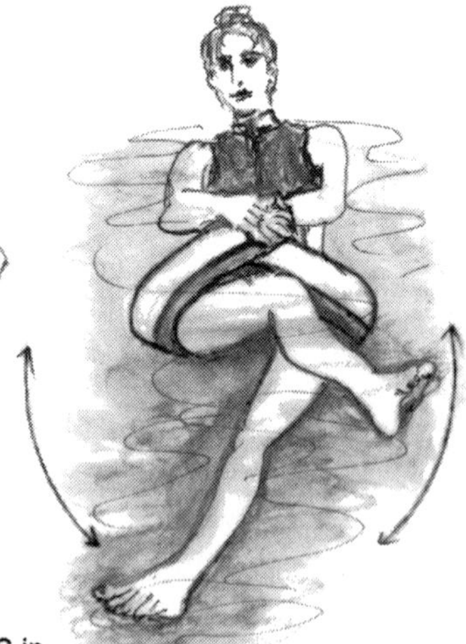

7) SITTING in
a SWING
c) scissors cross

AEROBIC NOODLING:

1) JOGGING FORWARD: in a more challenging variation of water walking than what's been previously described in the warm-up- place the noodle on the surface of the water directly in **front** of you with your arms draped over it -for more challenge, try resting your forearms on the noodle and pushing it down a few inches as you move forward-

2) JOGGING BACKWARD: pull the noodle around **behind** you, rest your arms on top of it and think of sitting down in a chair, the emphasis is now on bringing your knees up high, pulling the belly button up into the ribs and keeping the neck and shoulders as relaxed as possible while the water massages your back-

3) RIDING the HORSE: straddle a noodle (if you're not tall, you might prefer the shorter version of the athletic 'Sqoodle' from Aqua Jogger so it won't bop you in the back of your head), grab your dumbbells if you're strong, come to your usual depth of water and begin a big **jog** pushing the dumbbell down with the leg going down, focus on the propelled pushing off the bottom of the pool- keep that tummy tight-

4) CROSS COUNTRY SKI: (still straddling the noodle) now remaining **suspended** again think about jumping hurdles, trying to kick your buttocks with the heel in back and really punching the dumbbell out over the opposite leg in front- (a powerful kick and punch here will really carve out your core while giving a great cellulite massage to your legs!)

5) SCISSOR KICKS: (still straddling the noodle) bring the feet together on the bottom of the pool and push off the bottom, right leg going up in **front** and left leg going up in **back** for 8 counts, then switch to left in front and right going up in back, continue for counts of 4, 2's, and alternating singles- keep your grip on the dumbbells as relaxed as possible with the elbows soft -

6) WATER ANGEL: lift your legs and lean back making **a big sweeping motion** with the arms and the legs, **crossing the arms and legs** as you come back to center- point the toes out and dig the heels across, keeping the neck as relaxed as possible-

7) SITTING in a SWING: sounds like? Yes, **sit on the noodle** wrapping your hands about the ends, now keeping the knees slightly bent, **(a) kick alternating legs up in front** and press the opposite end of the noodle towards the knee that's coming up (be sure you're leaning forward a bit) -after 8-16 repetitions, switch to a **(b) scissors move** without touching bottom, if you're strong, cross alternating arms and legs **(c)**, pointing the toes out, digging the heels across and wrapping the ends of the noodle around your torso-

8) POGO JUMPS: beginning at the sides of the pool, **put one foot down on the middle of the noodle and then the other**, stay arms length from the side of the pool, keep your elbows slightly bent while gently griping the sides of the pool, begin jumping **on the noodle,** it helps you maintain balance if you push hard off the bottom of the pool -the goal is to move away from the sides of the pool and jump vigorously... for the very strong, try holding the ends of the noodle while jumping -

9) PUSH AWAYS: transitioning to a very relaxing move, stand (feet together) in chest deep water, clasping the middle of the noodle, hands shoulder width apart, now **push** vigorously off the bottom of the pool, simultaneously **pushing the noodle away** along the surface of the water- enjoy the water massage and allow the feet to drop naturally to the pool bottom, then reverse the direction and repeat ...

10) PUSH and PULLS: for the very *strong*, try this move without touching bottom: tuck the **knees to the noodle** and then **push away** vigorously with the arms and the legs, for an extra core challenge, tuck and kick repeatedly going in a circular direction and then reverse the circle-

YOGA AND PILATES inspired **noodling** moves include the following:

1) SIMPLE COBRA: vigorously pushing *off* the bottom of the pool, keeping the knees straight as the stretch will go deeper into the back (if it hurts the back, just bend the knees and you will come out of it) -allow the feet to drop naturally and repeat as desired, the water massage is great!

2) ADVANCED COBRA: this position can be had by placing the noodle across the waist and **pushing** *off* the bottom, make a big butterfly with the arms- focus on breathing and deep relaxation-

MAKING WAVES: USE YOUR NOODLE
YOGA & PILATES INSPIRED NOODLING

6) A NOODLING
FINISH

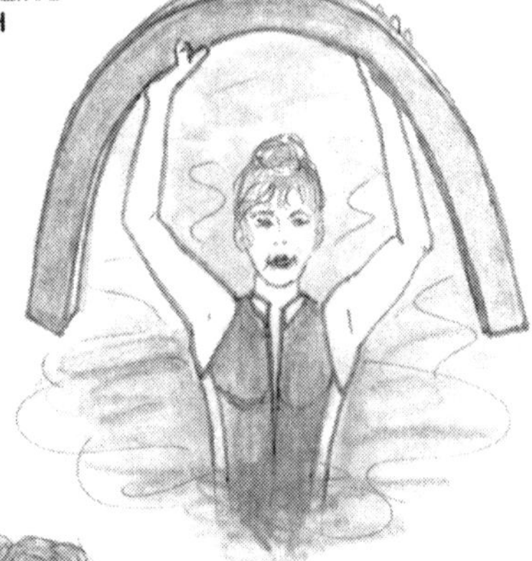

1,2) COBRA

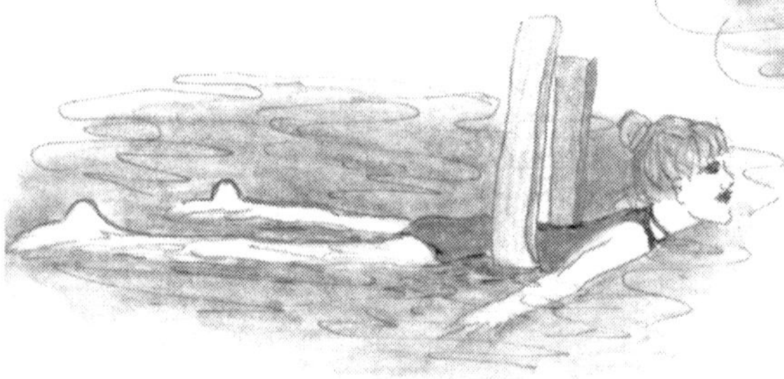

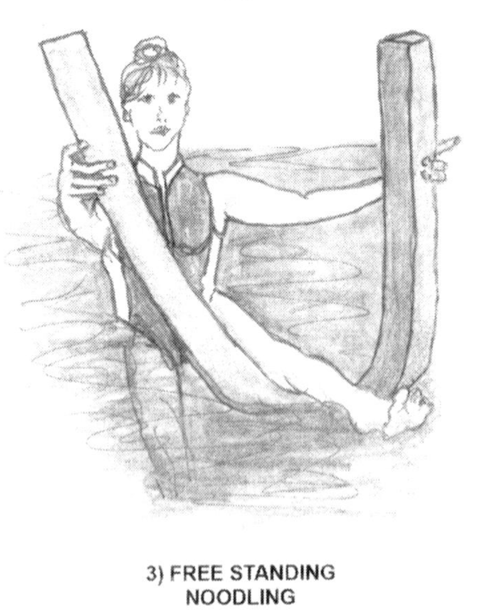

3) FREE STANDING
NOODLING

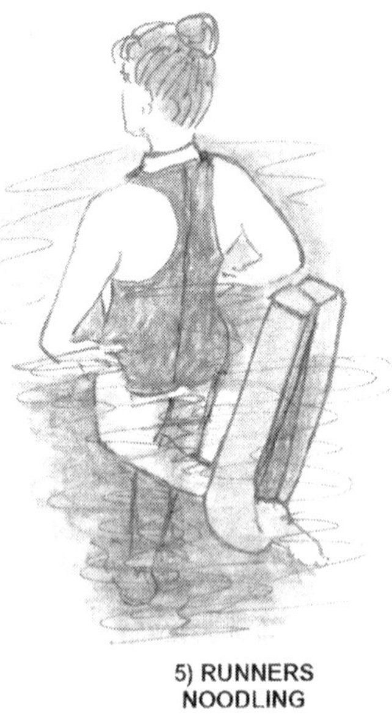

5) RUNNERS
NOODLING

3) FREE STANDING NOODLING: in waist to chest high water, lift the right leg, and place the **noodle just above the heel** of the right foot and **pull up** on the noodle, point and flex the foot, circle the ankle, then reverse the circle- (keep that standing leg slightly bent at the knee!)

4) NOODLING THIGHS: now **bringing both ends of the noodle together** with the right hand, swing the right leg, still on the noodle over to your right side, (keeping the standing left knee slightly bent for balance)-now **push down** through the heel of the right foot then **control** the upward motion as you return to the surface of the pool with a pointed toe (pull the belly button up higher into the ribs as you press down with the exhale)- 8x-

5) RUNNER'S NOODLING: next **bend the right knee** and swing it to the rear in a **runner's stretch** with the noodle under the top of the foot, keeping the knees together, and again holding a noodle end with each hand, **push down** with the top of the foot and then **control** the upward motion (stay centered in the core muscles and the breathing) - 8x-, (avoid these moves if you have joint issues)-

6) A NOODLE FINISH: holding the noodle with hands shoulder width apart, **reach** the long **arms straight up**, inhaling, then **press** the noodle to the **right** with an exhale- come back to **center** inhaling, then press **left** exhaling, back to **center** with an inhale- then bring the noodle to the **neck** pulling it gently and taking **right ear** to **right shoulder**, **left ear** to **left shoulder** with a slow exhale... (the cool damp noodle feels great here!)

7) RELAXATION POSE: resting the neck on one noodle and another noodle under the knees, breathe deeply and enjoy the weightless sensation of supported **floating**... if you love this, you are an excellent candidate for a **WATSU Treatment** with a water massage therapist or an assisted water stretch.

MAKING WAVES: GOING DEEP

"Can ye fathom the ocean, dark and deep,
where the mighty waves and the grandeur sweep?"
~ Fanny Crosby

"We ourselves feel that what we are doing
is just a drop in the ocean. But the ocean would be less
because of that missing drop."
~ Mother Teresa

Deep-water aquatic exercise is an unbeatable opportunity to unload the compressive forces on the spinal discs and joints resulting from body weight and gravity while simultaneously focusing on endurance and coordination. The vertical body works against 4x the resistance that is encountered in the usual horizontal swim position while benefitting from this subtle yet sustained traction. A **Floatation Device** such as the AquaJogger belt is a requirement for participation as it serves to foster and maintain a neutral spinal alignment. The hump on the belt faces the upper back and helps you maintain an erect posture as there is no bending at the waist; the entire body is leaning slightly forward. More athletic and seasoned participants may also enjoy using **leg cuffs** and choosing from a large assortment of **resistance tools** for the hands such as webbed gloves or plastic devices. If you choose to wear **aquatic exercise shoes**, these will also add resistance. See illustrations-

MAKING WAVES: GOING DEEP

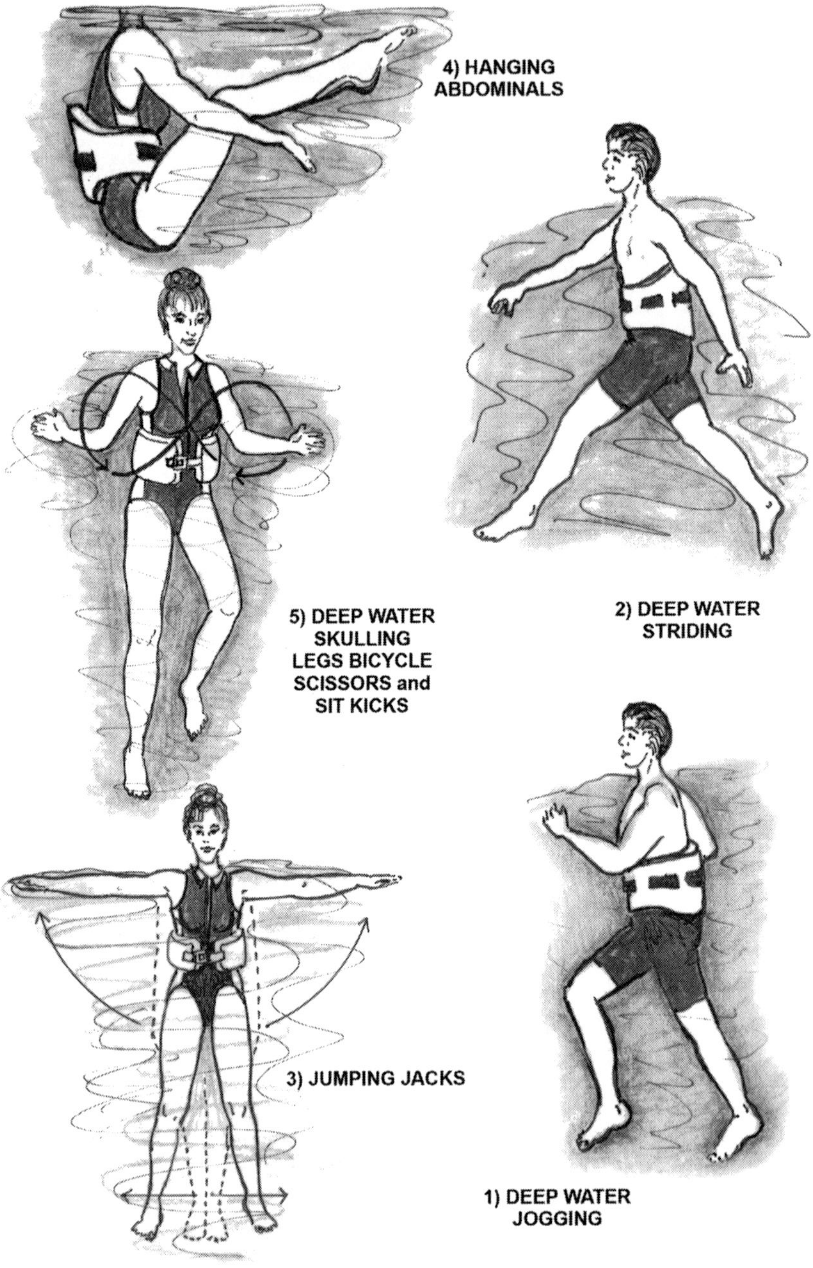

1) DEEP WATER JOGGING- this is the foundation of your deep water cardiovascular conditioning and should be progressively increased beginning with a 5-7 minute interval. Be certain that your waist belt has been tightly secured as it can feel looser and tend to ride up once you are exercising in the water. **Lean slightly forward** and begin jogging similarly to what you'd do on land (elbows at a 90-degree angle as you pump the arms and bicycle the legs) but be certain to **straighten the leg** out completely on the downward portion of the motion to further benefit from decompression.

2) STRIDING- leaning forward slightly as above, the elbows and knees remain locked in this motion that resembles a **stiff legged march**. As you swing the opposite arms and legs forward pull the foot up to flex the thigh muscles. Begin striding for 1-2 minutes, alternating with the longer intervals of water jogging. The faster you stride, the more resistance you will encounter from the water and you may need to shorten the stride.

3) JUMPING JACKS- with the waist belt secure as in all deep water exercise, perform the jumping jack bringing the **arms** just up near the surface of the water but not breaking the surface while pushing the **legs** open. This can be performed in intervals of 1-3 minutes. Variations such as adding a tuck or a more plyometric jack as described previously in the shallow water 'Splash Dance' sequence (II, 4) can be fun as can the addition of dumbbells-

4) HANGING ABDOMINALS- a pair of large **dumbbells** will help your maintain your balance (along with the waist belt) as you **lift both knees** up your midline **to the chest** and then control their downward motion. Next pull both knees up towards the **right armpit** (being certain to twist at the waist rather than the hips) and then control their downward motion. Repeat to the **left armpit** and then back to the mid chest. Gradually increase your repetitions to 1-2 minutes. If this puts too much stress on your shoulder joints, try dumbbells under the arms for support- Another technique for abdominals involves brining the feet and knees up over the edge of the pool and then supporting the back of the head with the fingertips (elbows open, careful to support the neck as opposed to pulling) as you lift the torso toward the knees and then lower it into the water. For the very strong, this is a fun variation of the usual land based sit-up-

5) SCULLING- is a good recovery technique to practice as a break from more intense intervals, begin with thumbs up and palms facing each other, turn the thumbs down as you move the hands down and away from the center of the body in a **figure eight motion.** It can be used with a **bicycle** motion of the legs, with **scissors**, or with **sit kicks**-

6) VIDEO CLIPS that feature deep water, see www.watergym.com where you can also purchase equipment and find classes or instructors-

MAKING WAVES: MORE DEPTH

"So many people spend their health gaining wealth,
and then have to spend their
wealth to regain their health"
~A.J. Reb Materi

"Those who do not find time for exercise
will have to find time for illness."
~ Earl of Derby

I have taken wonderful certification trainings with The Arthritis Foundation and The MS Society. If you have been diagnosed with either and you are reasonably fit, you can learn a great deal that will maximize your future quality of life in these trainings. For a beginning instructor, they are a very affordable means to acquire valuable knowledge that will help you understand the pain and suffering of many students/ clients and the most effective ways to help them with water exercise. Continuing education is a must for professionals and I *love* my AKWA Magazine, the official publication of the Aquatic Exercise Association- available at www.aeawave.com as is the definitive resource AQUATIC FITNESS PROFESSIONAL MANUAL, 6th edition. In addition, my personal library includes the following:

1) *THE COMPLETE WATERPOWER WORKOUT BOOK*, 1993 by Linda Huey and Robert Forster offers specialized training tips for athletes, dancers, as well as specific exercises for nonsurgical injuries.

2) *FANTASTIC WATER WORKOUTS,* 2nd edition- 2007 by MaryBeth Pappas Baun includes Yoga Booty Ballet and Country Line Dancing techniques as well as special needs-

3) *WATER EXERCISE:* 78 Safe and Effective Exercises for Fitness and Therapy, 1998 by Martha White

4) *YOUR WATER WORKOUT:* No-impact Aerobic and Strength Training From Yoga, Pilates, Tai Chi, and more, 2003, by Jane Katz

5) *THE NEW W.E.T. WORKOUT* by Jane Katz, 1996 offers a progressive twelve week program, in depth pregnancy fitness, and synchronized swimming-

6) *WATER FITNESS LESSON PLANS AND CHOREOGRAPHY,* 2010 by Christine Alexander is a terrific resource for instructors in training-

WHAT IS FUNCTIONAL FITNESS?

"Lack of activity destroys the
good condition of every human being,
while movement and methodical physical exercise
save it and preserve it."
~ Plato

"I find that making love is the best form of exercise."
~ Cary Grant

"If your dog is fat, you're not getting enough exercise."
~ Unknown

"Sex without love is merely healthy exercise."
~ Robert A. Heinlein

Sometimes at dinner parties or other potentially awkward social occasions, when I've had my limit of red wine, I love to tell my tale of a robbery gone wrong. "I had parked my car and was digging change out of my purse for the parking meter when suddenly a bicycle swopped past and my purse was snatched out of my hands. The thief was a teenaged boy gleefully racing up Robertson Blvd. I wasted no time in running after him. Up ahead at an intersection, I thought I saw a cop car and he must have seen the same because he suddenly spun around back toward me. He freaked out when he realized I was right on his tail! I had removed my jacket and I threw it at his head, suddenly the bike skidded onto its side and the little thief was sprawled across the pavement, struggling under the weight of the bicycle. I picked up my purse and jacket as he began screaming at me, "You f***ing bitch!" It was a pleasure to reply, "Shut your dirty mouth or I can have the cops here pronto!"

When I think of that recent fitness buzz phrase, 'Functional Fitness', I can't help but recall this incident and how great it felt to be able to take care of myself in that way. My idea of functional fitness is, in fact, based on the premise that I want to remain capable of running fast enough and long enough to escape my neighborhood zombies. I want to be able to swim well enough and long enough to flee from a shark and kick him with a resounding whack in the schnoz. I need to be able to lift heavy furniture, luggage, and I need the strength to continue teaching twelve hours weekly. Perhaps you're training for the Iron Man Triathlon and looking to strengthen your core without suffering repetitive motion wear-and-tear. Or maybe, you simply want to lift your grandchildren without throwing your back out. Whatever your needs may be, functional fitness addresses the idea that it is a group of muscles working together that you want to train as opposed to the old notion that you might wanna pump your biceps 'cause it looks good.

There are many new ideas being presented in gyms all over the country that support this notion that it can be more effective to work muscles in unison than it is to isolate them. It's almost amusing to me as a water exercise instructor because our muscles are nearly always working in unison in the water. The unique properties of water make it an ideal environment for rehabilitation from injuries. It also makes it an ideal training environment for the athlete who wants an edge in his game or sport. Overtraining is a thing of the past for the athlete who excels in a repetitive motion endeavor such as cycling, swimming, golf, tennis, football, etcetera, if he trains the opposing and supporting muscle groups in water. Not only are you getting the training, but you are also giving your joints some new life; what with the hydrostatic pressure and the lymphatic massage that naturally occurs.

"It's only exercise" is a phrase I'm fond of repeating because we have so much stress to deal with in this uncertain twenty-first century and exercise is such a great way to process that stress. We certainly don't need to be stressing over the de-stressor, exercise can be fun! How much exercise do we need? The U.S. government finally stepped up its recommendation to one hour daily. One hour sounds like a lot, but not when you consider that everything you do counts. You can break it up over the course of the day if need be. Take the stairs at work, walk the dog. Everything counts!

Some years ago, walking was all the rage because some study had been done which demonstrated the incredible jump in fitness that occurred when you get up off the couch and move; walking compared to *sedentarism*. If we were to discuss your optimal fitness level however, walking alone is insufficient. Don't get me wrong, it's all good, but in the interest of maximizing your time and health, I suggest you pick up some hand weights that slip around your wrists. That's a little **TRICK** that will bump your heart rate up a bit more and you'll barely notice the increased exertion as you walk.

On the other hand, the closer you get to your optimal fitness level, the harder you will be working. What you may not be able to imagine is just how good it feels to be functioning at that level. There are endorphin highs to be had when you show up as your fittest self and work to maintain what you've earned. You simply won't know how good you can feel until you try.

Since there are limits to what I can explore in this volume, I'd like to introduce you to a few **TIPS** for at home fitness maintenance that really work for me and my clients:

1) **LIFT A LITTLE:** Busy people can't always make it to the gym for a class but you can certainly keep a few free weights at your home or office. It's good thinking to turn your children on to a fitness habit or even inspire your spouse. Lifting light to medium-heavy weights and going quickly from one exercise to another continues to show up in studies as being most efficacious. If you're female, and you worry about building bulky muscle; sticking to very light weight, you may wanna rethink that because you're missing the opportunity to maximize your metabolism. What looks 'bulky' now, may simply be your remaining body fat, which will continue to diminish over time as you work at it. A good trainer can be instrumental in inspiring you to continue on until you meet your goals. I've added some kettlebell exercises to my routines as it challenges the core and gets the heart rate up higher for my busy clients needing to maximize their time. When they coined the phrase "Use it or Lose it", they knew what they were talking about. It has been demonstrated in a years long study that joints which are exercised consistently will outlast and outperform the joints of the sedentary. Least we forget, muscle mass burns calories even when we sleep!

2) HAVE A BALL: The fitness ball gets my vote as one of the best items to hit the market *big* time, and for good reason. It's a fun and versatile item which I can't imagine not having. Did I mention that I'm sitting on one right now at my computer? (Sitting on it forces core recruitment!) It comes in three sizes: 55, 65, and 75 cm. Its very presence in a room invites you to play! Usually, there is a DVD included but YouTube can give you some good exercises as well. I like to end my sculpting classes with a seated bounce on the ball "Lift the arms overhead and then hit the ball, eight will do, then give me some punches, then overhead again, now counts of four..." Did you know that bouncing stimulates your lymphatic system? Too bad you gave away that old mini trampoline.

3) ROCK AND ROLL: The roller log keeps evolving and what was a hard white styrofoam cylinder has become a softer blue or black model. I found a cheap version at my local discount store that is a blow up cylinder (like the fitness ball and so pretty too). It actually gives you an opportunity for a good core workout as you roll away your aches and pains. Some supervision to learn how to use it is very helpful, but again, there are video's available.

4) UPSIDE DOWN: I have an inversion machine in my living room, am I a freak or what? In my case, it's an occupational necessity. I often teach an aquatics class first thing in the morning, followed by a cycling class, followed by some lifting... You get the picture. Would that it were the other way around, but my inversion table can fold up and disappear when I don't need it to unload my spine at the end of the day. It's not for everybody as my friends' trials and tribulations on mine have taught me. But, if you're a reasonably fit person who isn't dealing with blood pressure issues, you just might love it too.

5) DRY BRUSH MASSAGE: Clients and friends who have lost a good deal of weight will often complain of hanging skin and this technique is a sure way to increase circulation and lymphatic drainage while improving skin tone. Once you begin to enjoy the sensation and benefits, you will never want to risk your good dry brush getting wet in the bath again, other than for periodic cleaning. On a day when I have time, I like to sit on a stool and begin at the bottom of my feet, moving upwards towards the heart in a firm little circular motion. I do this with a hand sized brush and then I later stand and use a long handled brush to reach tough areas of the back. It feels wonderfully relaxing and indulgent but it also gives a terrific boost to our bodies second organ of elimination...

6) PURSUE YOUR PASSION: You adults may already have found pleasure in sports and athletic pursuits, and that may be one reason why you need aquatic exercise now. Years ago, we were clueless about stretching. When we finally discovered it's benefits, we failed to advise people that they needed to get their core muscles warm before pushing those stretches. We keep learning new information. I was fortunate to have an hour of gym class everyday in grade school, though I hated it at the time. Today's girls have so many more options and opportunities to see themselves as feminine and fit. Boy's, I would think of as a no brainer for athletic activities but unfortunately many are sucked into video games and the pressure to excel in academics. Also, in this economy, many kids need help to get an opportunity for their athletic development and in achieving a healthier diet. If you can help, there are many organizations in need of volunteers, and it can be incredibly rewarding to help children find their passion.

FITNESS FACTOIDS

"Our business in life is not to get ahead of others,
but to get ahead of ourselves- to break our own records,
to outstrip our yesterday by our today."
~ Stewart B. Johnson

"My invitation to you is to begin living every moment
as though you are miraculous and deserve to live an
extraordinary life. Fake it if you must and keep faking it
until it is real to you. The gift you will be giving yourself
is a lifelong journey of discovery, one that is infinite and
infinitely rewarding. Begin the journey.
Today. This moment. Now."
~ Robert White

"You learn you can do your best even when it's hard,
even when you're tired and maybe hurting a little.
It feels good to show some courage."
~ Joe Namath

I figure I will do almost daily aerobic cardiorespiratory training and work the intervals hard, approaching my maximum heart rate repeatedly, engage in free weight training at least two or three times weekly, or combine the two in a vigorous, refreshing aquatic exercise class, and I will be on my way... fortunately for me, I still get paid for doing this. Fortunately for you, there are many terrific instructors who take great pride in providing you a fun, upbeat, and effective workout that will do all these things for you. I had my favorite classes and favorite instructors that I frequented before I became one and someday, if I stop teaching, I will again attend classes. I admit that I can be a wimp. I can be very lazy but it doesn't make me feel good later. I need my classes and I need you to come join me. It's my job to motivate you but your attendance motivates me also. Somehow, a large class bumps it up a notch.

I also figure I will burn as many calories as possible by creating more metabolically active muscle tissue. In turn, I will be able to eat as much as I like of the good carbs: the vegetables, fruits, and some whole grains. The body cannot store carbohydrates; reserves are depleted in six hours. The other carbs, the 'bad' ones, are the ones I used to crave like a madwoman, occasionally, still do. When I'm feeling really good, they present very little temptation. When I consume lot's of organic brightly colored produce, I like knowing that I'm giving my body a great opportunity to process all these phytonutrients for the sake of healing and renewal. There is oxidative distress as a result of exercise (as a result of many other things also!) and these precious antioxidants that protect the plant will do the job for us as well. Frequently, I think of myself as being my own little science project.

Dr. Carson Chow, of The National Institute of Health is a mathematician who has applied his gifts to the study of obesity. He says there is clear experimental evidence that caloric intake beyond energy expenditure will lead to excess body weight and fat. For him, 'what we weigh' is a mathematical model based on the things we understand about metabolism. He says, "The metabolic cost of muscle is much higher than the metabolic cost of fat. The more you exercise, the faster you can get to steady state. All diets work but change takes a very long time, a year or more." According to his research, "food availability has increased since the mid-nineteen-seventies to an additional one thousand calories per person...progressively wasting more food per person, per day." He postulates that the availability of fast, cheap, and massive foodstuffs has fueled the obesity epidemic. If you go online to www.bwsimulator.niddk.nih.gov., you can post your information and you will discover how much you will need to reduce your intake and increase your activity to lose weight. Also, the length of time required to reach your goal.

While researching Dr. Chow, I came across his online correspondence with Dr. William L. Wilson of the CARB Syndrome Project. Dr. Wilson emphasizes the idea that diet composition plays a key role in determining body composition. "I have measured the body composition of many women with pre-terminal anorexia and they always have some degree of excessive body fat in relationship to their lean body mass- this certainly cannot be explained by excessive calories. When these women do eat, it's almost always food containing sucrose, HFCS (High Fructose Corn Syrup), and high glycemic carbohydrates. When auto-regulating functions are intact, short term over-feeding doesn't appear to lead to significant fat storage. When these functions are disrupted by consuming foods containing excess fructose and high glycemic carbohydrates, fat storage tends to occur even if lean body mass is lost by under-eating. That's how you end up with an obese thin person."

I credit Dr. Mark Hyman, author of "THE BLOOD SUGAR SOLUTION" with bringing the term 'diabesity' into mainstream consciousness. You can go to www.drhyman.com. and take his free Ultra Wellness Quiz which will help you determine your risk for this condition that is almost never treated directly as there is no drug to prescribe for it. It is, however, the hidden cause of heart disease, hypertension, high cholesterol, stroke, dementia, many cancers (breast, colon, prostate, pancreatic, liver, and kidney), and even depression. Dr.Hyman offers articles and recipes in his efforts to 'upgrade our biological software'. The website also provides an opportunity for professionals to come together in the study and practice of 'Functional' medicine.

There are costly tests, body scans and MRIs which can determine with accuracy the degree of abdominal obesity someone may have, but honestly, you can bet your big belly you've got it. Clinicians wanting to use simple science to prove it to you will often refer to the **Body Mass Index (BMI)** which is determined by computing a number based on the height and weight of an individual. Using the formula for BMI, let's look at the statistics for a 5 foot-5 inches tall female who weighs 140 pounds.

1) weight = 140 pounds
2) divided by your height in inches square
65 x 65 = 4225 (140 / 4225 = 0.033)
3) 0.033 x 703 = **23.3 Your Body Mass Index**
(she would be considered normal)

BODY MASS INDEX FORMULA

1) Body Weight In Pounds
2) Divided By Your Height In Inches Squared
3) Multiplied By 703

BODY MASS INDEX RESULTS

1) Below 18.5------------------ Underweight
2) 18.5 - 24.9 ------------------ Normal Range
3) 25.0 - 29.9 ------------------ Overweight
4) 30.0 and Above ----------- Obese

Critics claim that the **BMI** fails to differentiate between body mass from fat and body mass from muscle. If you are among the generally inactive population and your number is 25 or higher, you would be wise to begin a dedicated attempt at lowering this number. On the other hand, if you are an elite athlete, this can be quite inaccurate. Shaquille O'Neal, arguably one of the all-time best NBA stars was 'obese' at 7' 1" and 320 pounds. At the time, few professionals would consider 'obesity' to be an accurate assessment of his condition. For this reason, BMI should generally not be the sole diagnostic tool for determining health risks...

The **WHR** or **Waist-Hip Ratio** measurement may be a more accurate tool for risk assessment as it considers the consequences of fat distribution. The 'apple' body shapes are at greater risk than the 'pear' shapes, which carry the weight in the hips as opposed to the stomach. According to "TIME MAGAZINE", people who are pear shaped have a less aggressive insulin response and therefore experience less fluctuation in the blood sugar that leads to over eating. Of course, this does not mean that you don't have a problem with excess fat. It just means that your body responds differently to diet and exercise than the apple shape. If the looking glass leaves you mystified about your shape, here is the formula:

CALCULATING WAIST-HIP RATIO

1) Measure your waist circumference at the belly button. Hold the tape measure straight.
2) Measure your hips at the widest point, where the buttocks peak.
3) Divide your waist measurement by your hip measurement.

Using the Waist-Hip-Ratio, risk is rated by how high the numbers are. For women, the higher the number past 0.8, the greater the risk of obesity related disorders. For example, using the 'ideal' of 0.8 or less - a female with a 29" waist and 36" hips just makes the cutoff. For men, anything over .95 indicates increased risk. A man with 34" waist and 36" hips would represent the 'ideal'.

Obesity is perhaps the most obvious risk factor in Metabolic Syndrome. Keep in mind, however, that increasing age, a family history of diabetes, hormonal imbalance, and even race, as well as an unhealthy lifestyle are potential contributing factors in addition to insulin resistance. The good news however, is that these factors are very responsive to a comprehensive upgrade in our daily habits, one that includes regular exercise as being most efficacious in mitigating these associated risks....

SPINDERELLA RIDES AGAIN, and AGAIN, and AGAIN...

"My idea of exercise is a good brisk sit"
~ Phyllis Diller

"Motivation is what gets you started,
habit is what keeps you going"
~ Jim Ryun

"Sit on your butt and do something."
~ Mountain biking shirt

On behalf of the growing legions of 'SPINSTERS', devout indoor cyclists who have found a way to have their cake and eat it too, I must admit that I am a devote. Four times a week I lead a class in indoor cycling, I go to great lengths to prepare new and exciting playlists and I don't seem to tire of it-- ever! There is just something about the loud music (I call my music loud when I've been known to wear ear plugs at another instructors class!), the camaraderie, the endorphin high, the lack of wear and tear on the joints...just something downright *sexy* about spin. That's not to mention the sexy looking 'behind' that will do your best jeans proud.

Now, least we forget to mention it, it was the infamous Johnny G (AKA Jonathan Goldberg) who back in nineteen eighty-six decided it was a concept worth exploring, this indoor cycling business. Mr. Goldberg has a very colorful history, the son of a South African pharmacist who trained in the gym above his father's pharmacy. He first came to Los Angeles in nineteen seventy-nine only to be robbed of his three thousand dollar savings on the third day he was here. Apparently a resourceful fellow from the start, he managed to persuade a Venice gym to give him a shot at personal training. In the following decade, he earned a black belt in martial arts and became a competitive bicycle racer; twice competing in cross-country races. In thinking to create an indoor training system for himself, he launched 'Madd Dog Athletics' and within two years found a successful home at Voight Fitness in West Hollywood.

Today there are many names and variations (as well as trademarks!) that have sprung from Johnny G's baby but fans like myself want him to know we feel a debt of gratitude. In a typical forty minute class you can expect to burn from four hundred to nine hundred calories and your furnace will be pumped for the remainder of the day. You may recall that burning thirty-five hundred stored calories will result in the loss of one pound, so you can see that a regular 'spinster' has a method to her madness. There's that and there's also a great opportunity to vent your frustrations in a healthy manner.

When you're a newbie to my classes (and to indoor cycling in general), it's always good to arrive ten minutes early so that I can give you a little personal attention. It works equally well for me if you stop in after a class and introduce yourself. This gives me an opportunity to help you learn to adjust the bike. I prefer the seat a little lower than some people, I believe it helps you recruit the muscles around the knees and strengthen them as you come up out of the saddle. However, the seat is never so low as to turn your knees out to the sides when seated. There are only a few positions to learn on the bike coupled with the variations in resistance that result in 'hills' and 'sprints' and 'slides".

Sounds easy? It can actually be quite frustrating in the beginning... athletes from other sports often wonder 'WTF' when they attempt lot's of jumps and find it more challenging than previously imagined. The moves on a bike are what we call 'sport specific', your prowess at tennis, running, or swimming will not necessarily make those jumps any easier as they require the use of 'fast twitch' muscle fiber. Unless you are genetically gifted, it usually requires three or more months of regular participation to grow that muscle.

Like most women who take up indoor cycling, I was very concerned that I not build large bulky thigh muscle in the process. What worked for me was a focus on sprints with light resistance and not so much emphasis on hills with maximum resistance. I'm always amused by the fact that men seem to like quite the reverse; in fact, many men seem to particularly hate jumps with light resistance. Now that I've been instructing for years, it doesn't seem to matter much what I do (my body seems to stay the same)... so I try to gear my class towards those in attendance. I encourage first timers to do as much time as possible and don't worry about the fancy stuff. I would prefer to see you come back and work a little harder every few days than to imagine you're cursing me behind my back because of your aching butt!

Smart-ass that I tend to be, I must confess (always I'm confessing in these pages!) That I waited a year after I began teaching before I broke down and splurged on some shoes. What a fool I was! The shoes make the work so much more fun because your feet are connected to the pedals. If indoor cycling will be the only time you use the shoes, they certainly don't need to be expensive. There are many great deals available and you can also find them online. As for other gear, I prefer spandex tights that hit just below the knee, the kind with built in diaper 'cush' are an unfortunate look; better and cheaper to buy a bike seat cushion. I like a racer back "T" because I will get quite sweaty... and a water bottle is a real necessity.

Like many who've been cycling for some years, it always seemed to me like it would be worth trying to do something *more* with the upper body in the process. All the latest research showed me that we would burn significantly more calories by riding for one-half hour, getting off the bike to do some opposing muscle work with weights and then getting back on the bike for another half hour. During the first and second segments on the bike, I have incorporated some lightweight work that we do while riding seated, with moderately heavy resistance on a couple 'hill' songs. It seems to be a very effective workout. I am certainly exhausted when finished but I was shocked when Joe took my class two weeks in a row and showed me the results on his new Polar Heart Rate monitor... I sent them off an e-mail at Polar asking "seriously, is that even possible?" and their reply was to make sure the electrodes which contact the skin are cleaned regularly... Go figure!

Now, I am very careful to be sure the core muscles are well engaged when we add the weights and I make certain my participants are seasoned spinners, with no back pain, coming into class. I have read about such classes where there seems to be more risk- or at least they found a couple fitness experts who talked it down as dangerous. It amuses me a little because I think dangerous compared to what? We who love our sports will always be seeking more challenge and variety...

Before wrapping up this little chapter, I think it fair to warn you ladies that when I say spin classes can be sexy, I'm not joking... I feel compelled to inform you that there can be a lot of 'musical chair' type games going on with the sharing of sexual partners, at least in the hot classes of big cities...so beware and don't let a little flirtation lure you into something you might regret. Now you guys, it's a different matter... get thee to a spin class and you will never have to troll the bars or Internet again!

SAVING FACE

"You cannot save your ass and your face at the same time."
~ James Dowler Gow

"Youth is a gift of nature but age is a work of art."
~ Stanislow Jerzy Lec

"I'm tired of all this nonsense about beauty
being only skin-deep. That's deep enough.
What do you want, an adorable pancreas?"
~ Jean Kerr

"A man's face is his autobiography,
a woman's face is her work of fiction."
~ Oscar Wilde

Living in Los Angeles can be a daunting experience for the insecure, especially to those who make their living (or strive to) in show business. Almost always there is someone younger and better looking who can do the job, and generally speaking, they do.

I attended a showbiz seminar for women years ago where a very famous producer, Jay Bernstein, tickled us all with his comments. "Every unattractive little man in the world dreams of becoming a Hollywood producer so that he can sleep with beautiful women..." From my own experiences, I would say that it's also like the old Groucho Marx line "I wouldn't want to be a member of any club that would have me as a member". You are damned if you do and damned if you don't as long as your self-esteem is dependent on something external.

Since casting is first of all defined by 'externals' as described in the script breakdown, it can be a very nasty process. One has only to look online or in the tabloids, or tabloid style TV shows to see all the unfortunate mistakes made particularly (but not exclusively) by actresses seeking to make themselves more marketable. So often, it's the working actress, the ingénue with a 'certain spark' who succumbs to insecurity and goes for 'the works'. Unfortunately, when youth and beauty are combined with these procedures, the result is often a cartoon version of their former self.

I know personally how difficult it is to be told, "get a boob job" (when a series regular part went to what they all agreed was a less talented actress whose knockers bedazzled) when my boobs were quite 'spectacular' in my own estimation. "Too tall, too short, too fat, too old..." you will hear it all at one time or another. But wait, you may never hear 'too thin'... at least that was the case on a soap opera where it was rumored that a trainer refused to train a particular star for fear of anorexic heart failure. As long as the face looked good (and the bones can protrude so beautifully in a young face) -- there was no possibility of too thin.

That said, there does come a time for those who have had the pleasure and benefits of good looks, when they look in the mirror and all they see is 'sad sacks'. Disappointment with ones appearance can lead to insecurity and self-obsession and so a vicious cycle begins. But wait, before you indulge in the 'knifestyles of the rich and famous', let me share with you what I've experienced and what seems to work short of surgery. I'm certainly not against surgical solutions. I truly believe that anyone who suffers from the notion that one particular feature of their appearance is a roadblock to their success in life or to their attainment of love and happiness should address that feature. After all, you don't gain anything from 'blaming it' on the nose (or whatever) if your real problem is narcissism! These are among the many issues which I feel can benefit from short-term therapy. It's better not to drive your friends crazy (with these potentially obsessive thoughts) because a real friend loves you as you are... and your best friends won't hate you 'cause you're beautiful.

Least you think it's easy for me to dish this out, I admit that eventually I will perhaps invest in a little nip and tuck. It comes with a nice long rest and some powerful painkillers, which may be part of the attraction for women (and some men) of a certain age. An opportunity to reinvent yourself! Here in Tinsel Town, that 'certain age' can come at most any age. I've heard of actresses as young as twenty-eight getting a lift. It seems to me that there must be some features that were getting a little correction at such a young age, but what do I know?

I have tried most of the electric muscle stimulating home machines on the market. Either I purchased it or I borrowed a friend's to give it a try. All I can say is maintenance, maintenance, *maintenance...* (we may need the surgical downtime just to recover from maintenance!). I like the improvements I see around my eyes when I've used the Suzanne Summers model but it doesn't seem like a strong enough contraction around my jaw line to get results that are worth the time that must be invested there on a regular basis.

What does work wonders for me is more good old-fashioned *exercise*! I put together a series of eight exercises that make a huge difference for my facial structure in that my features appear to be more lifted and happy looking. There is more tautness in my neckline, definition in my chin, and lift to my eyes. I admit that despite owning a couple books devoted to facial exercise (and some darned expensive equipment!), what works best for me are these simple exercises that I learned from books as well as videos on the Internet... *FOR FREE!* Best of all, though the initial learning curve is a tiny bit tedious, after you connect and really start to see and feel the difference in your face, you will no longer have to sit at your computer monitor or even in front of a mirror. Now you can use that wasteland of time spent stopped at red lights to scare the nearby drivers! It's also a great opportunity for multitasking long phone calls or watching sucky reality TV.

I do believe that with just a little filler in the hollows under my eyes (when I get the nerve!), I will be good to go for a while longer. After all, advantages to regular exercise of the body include superior skin tone as well as suppleness and elasticity. The exception to this, of course, is joggers... I have read and seen how the impact affects the face (not to mention the uterus, etc.) and all I can say is " bring that jogging to the water!"

Since I mentioned the subject of fillers, please bear with me here while I complain that some restraint needs to be instilled into the esthetic sensibilities of our culture. A puffy fat face used to be the result of drinking and drugs. While it's true that a little bit of filler in just the right area can perform miracles, too much is rather a horrifying look (and lately, we see it all the time!). Keep in mind that this kind of procedure is easy money for the doctor. It's so easy to get you in and out while the Doc plans his or her next vacation. Keep in mind also, that these products received FDA approval with very little time investment in studies. I plan to check out the new filler that is produced from a tiny piece of my own skin. Before moving on here, I feel compelled to suggest that all the Botox going into our faces is another gray area. The results may look nice but the coming years could prove there is a price to pay... One thing I do rave about is treatments like the LPL photo facial and other newer methods that actually stimulate collagen production while shrinking pores and eliminating fine lines and wrinkles. Nice!

Now, before getting started with my little series of facial exercises, I'd like to make it clear to you that it is my intention to make this fitness book of mine one of the best health and beauty bargains that you've ever invested in. In keeping with that promise, I am including an amazing skin treatment that will follow the exercises.

FACIAL EXERCISE PREPARATION:

1) Before you begin the exercises, It is important that you clean your face with a cream style facial cleanser. To prepare your own with ingredients you may already have on hand, try a teaspoon of organic mayonnaise or prepare the following-

Milky Cleanser: in a small clean glass jar, mix 2 parts full fat yogurt or cream with one part coconut, almond, or jojoba oil. Add 2 teaspoons of raw honey as it is a natural humectant (helping the skin retain moisture), and antibacterial, add 2 teaspoons of ground oatmeal or flaxseed meal-

Oily Skin Cleanser: in a small glass blender jar or mortar and pestle, place 3-5 very ripe organic strawberries, 2 teaspoons raw honey, adding sufficient ground oatmeal to thicken with a drop or 2 of an essential oil such as lavender or rose.

I suggest applying a good moisturizer around the eye area as you will want to be certain you are not aiding the formation of new wrinkles in your attempts to retain or regain a more youthful appearance.

2) It's very helpful to be **Seated** at a desk or table with your computer screen and / or **Mirror** at eye level. When I say computer screen, it's only necessary If you'd like to see demonstrations of these and other exercises on YouTube. Hopefully, these descriptions will be adequate but it's a great resource if you have facial issues that I fail to address here.

GETTING STARTED WITH FACIAL EXERCISES:

1) BOTTI: Think of Chris Botti as trumpeters tend to have very firm cheeks. That said, imitation can be flattering- to us. Fill the cheeks with air and attempt to shift the air from one cheek to the other, back and forth. At first this was difficult for me, but it definitely gets easier with practice... now I can do variations, I'll call them little 'pulses' that work on the nasal labial area and relax the corners of the mouth.

2) PROM QUEEN: Open the mouth and the eyes as widely as possible. Try to feel what's happening to the muscles around your ears and temples. With practice you can wiggle the ears by adding a slight smiley lift of the cheeks...

3) FISH FACE: Suck in your cheeks until your lips purse out and you look ridiculous! Now smile and look more ridiculous... but you can feel that lifting action, can you not?

4) FINGER FLEX: Place the index fingers into your mouth, inside your cheeks, use your finger pads to pull the cheeks open and then flex the muscles to pull them back together. As with most exercises, 15 or so reps 2 x daily is a good number to aim for.

5) BROW LIFT: Resting your elbows on the desk or table, place your fingertips under the eyebrows and press upward gently. Simultaneously, try and pull your forehead down.

6) KISSING THE SKY: Sitting tall, head lifted, shoulders down...look straight upward toward the ceiling, while pursing the lips to kiss the sky, push your tongue up to the roof of your mouth (you will feel a slight burning sensation in your neck as if tightening the skin of a drum). Do this again and turn to your right slightly followed by another attempt looking toward your left this time. Repeat once more looking straight up and you will probably need a break from the burning sensation. Try to repeat again when cleansing your face...

Notes on Facial Exercise: At first it will seem like a large commitment of time and energy to analyze your needs objectively, to experiment with various exercises and determine what may be beneficial to your facial structure. After experimenting for a couple hours, I put together the above routine for myself. I was pleased to think that it might work when I performed enough repetitions to experience some soreness the next day. I was even more pleased to see apparent improvements after a couple weeks of doing this series every other day. I was thrilled when the cleft in my chin reappeared after some years absence. Now, I have it down to a routine like my other workouts. Seriously, I do perform 'Botti', 'Fish Face', and 'Prom Queen' while driving around town. This is a most effective use of the time where I often find myself scowling and cursing at traffic. And now, for the promised treatment...

GREATEST BEAUTY SECRET:

It's often been speculated that men seem to age less dramatically than women. I believe this may be due, in part, to their larger adrenal glands giving them a greater tolerance to stress. It may also be due to their having skin that is thirty percent thicker than women's as well as having thirty percent more oil glands in the skin. Perhaps you've heard beauty experts joke that men's often superior skin aging is due to their ritual of shaving. The ancient Egyptians recorded such use of a blade to scrape off dead skin as a health ritual and this may have been practiced by the Sumerians before them. Since the reproduction of new skin cells slows down by approximately ten days per decade, scraping off the thickening uppermost epidermis has two benefits. First of all, it eliminates the dullness that characterizes older skin, and secondly, it prompts more rapid cellular repair causing it to replicate the efficient twenty-one day turnaround of young skin. The following is a very good method to use between facial treatments and can even benefit men if they learn to Dry Exfoliate their forehead. With the exception of skin conditions such as acne and rosacea, most complexions can benefit from the enhanced penetration of products that this technique allows as well as a lustrous glow. Below is a breakdown of the treatment plus the items you'll need to get started. It may seem a little difficult in the beginning as you must approach this method cautiously and carefully observe the results on your own skin. However, with systematic practice, I hope you'll be as pleased with the results as I am.

1) A **Milky cleanser**, a necessity for removing any pigment based product including those that are oil free. A **Foamy Cleanser** can follow this if your skin is looking a little oily. If the skin is very dry, repeat the milky cleanser a second time. A warm wet **Washcloth** is necessity for removing both the first and the second cleansing from the face or the remaining residue will interfere with the effectiveness of your treatment.

2) Now a little mixture of **Dish Detergent** and **Baking Soda** is combined as your facial scrub. It sounds gross, I know, but there is a method to the madness as the alkalinity of this mixture will promote oil production as the skin tries to neutralize itself back to acidic. You want this increased oil production beneath the dead skin layers that will be coming off.

3) Take a small amount of **Talc** into your hands and massage the complexion. This will soothe and sedate the skin a bit after the harsh chemicals of the scrub. It will also provide 'slip' to a **Disposable Razor** and the **Tinkle Razor.** (I get mine at the 99-cent store here in LA where you can also find a small10x magnifying mirror with suction cups.)

4) Now sitting at a **Magnifying Mirror** with good light, use the disposable razor to remove any hair from the face. Next, take the Tinkle Razor in your dominant hand and holding tautly an area of about one square inch of skin between your thumb and fingers, maneuver the Tinkle at a 45 to 90 degree angle and 'plane' the skin. You may need to gesture and position your tongue inside the mouth to isolate an area. Pay special attention wherever you see the unfortunate consequences of aging such as fine lines, wrinkling, and discoloration. If you see no visible lifting of skin cells, try working from another direction being careful not to over do it and abrade the skin. If this sounds intimidating, look closely at the Tinkle, try it on your arm and you will see that you have to carefully work at it, it is certainly not scalpel sharp.

5) There is no need to worry that removing fine downy **Facial Hair** will cause it to turn into beard stubble, though these little hairs will be the victim of this process. If this ritual is performed weekly or bi monthly, there should be no cause for concern...

6) Now you can stroke your face and see the difference in texture as well as the diminished appearance of fine lines and wrinkles. You may want to mix a small amount of **Hydrocortisone** cream with your moisturizer but it is recommended that you avoid the application of stronger products for 24 hours. Sunscreen (chemical free) and make up may be applied if you're heading out doors.

7) Now is the time to pick up your phone and make an appointment with your **Dermatologist** if you're over due or you saw something in the above process to give you pause.

8) You can find this **Procedure** described in more detail (I am giving a simpler, personalized explanation here that has delivered big time benefits to my skin) online at: www. HowAll.Info- How to Avoid Plastic Surgery. The writer, a very experienced esthetician, says to "put $200 in your piggy bank every time you give yourself this treatment as it is Microdermabrasion and Dermaplaning in one". She advises to "begin your first treatment when you are not rushed as it has a learning curve of 3x. TAKE YOUR TIME, PAY ATTENTION, to what you are doing. Be careful around the eyebrows! Prepare to be carded when you go out!"

9) I was privileged many years ago to have a **Treatment** with a renowned Beverly Hills dermatologist named Theodore Sutnick. He was famous for supposedly treating Barbara Streisand and many other Hollywood beauties at the time and this was his method. "Put your tongue right there and don't move your tongue until I tell you to or you'll be sorry!" He finished up the scalpel scraping process with extractions and dry ice burns... we looked like a pizza face for a week and paid big bucks for this beauty ritual which can be yours now. (Minus dry ice burns, thank you very much!)

DIET… WHAT DIET?

"Do not reward yourself with food. You are not a dog."
~ Unknown

"If you can't control your peanut butter,
you can't expect to control your life."
~ Calvin and Hobbes

"Nothing will benefit human health and increase the
chances for survival on Earth as much as
the evolution to a vegetarian diet."
~ Albert Einstein

I promised you no diet ever again. But first, we must consider that the word diet had its first known use in the thirteenth century. From the Latin, *diaeta,* or the Greek, *diaita*, it's literal meaning was 'manner of living' or from *diaitasthai*, 'to lead one's life'. Modern usage of the word describes food and drink that is regularly provided or consumed, habitual nourishment, and or limited or punishing regimens designed to reduce weight.

Personally, I like the original usage and I encourage you to think in terms of how you choose to lead your life. In reality, we are always, and have always been, on a diet. However, that diet may be what was chosen for you by your parents and their parents before them, our environmental conditioning, so to speak. When it comes to eating, what we learn to like and feel comfortable with from our families can go back generations. The foods that were available during and after wars and famines generated strong emotional eating habits in our ancestors. Perhaps even more so, the late twentieth century 'affluenza' which brought us to our knees (to our current girth would be more accurate) as an unhealthy society captivated by prettily packaged faux foods with an abundance of salt, preservatives, conditioners and colorings, refined sugars and trans fats, the likes of which were nowhere to be found in nature.

HBO recently ran their devastating two part series, *THE WEIGHT OF THE NATION*. At one point, it was stated: "No publishing company would publish a book that said 'eat a little less, and move a little more'." Damn, I thought, that was precisely what I had in mind for you! The point being, it matters very much how you move a little more just as it matters very much how you choose to eat a little less.

In actuality, I eat quite a lot of food and you may be able to also- after you break your addictions to the sugars, salts, bad fats and refined carbohydrates as well as all the 'frankenfoods' packaged and preserved with chemical additives. These things are destroying our health and leaving us wide open to "diabesity, cancer, arthritis, Alzheimer's, and too many other diseases to name. In fact, recent research leads many to believe that the *kind* of calories we consume is more significant than their number alone. It seems much more than coincidence that the beginnings of the obesity epidemic coincided with the introduction of these junk food ingredients as well as the revised 'diet' plans that appeared around nineteen seventy seven. Some say that our nation has been the victim of 'bad science'. If your scale won't budge, perhaps you need to take inventory.

The father of modern nutrition, Dr. Henry Bieler, demonstrated in his own practice that *FOOD IS YOUR BEST MEDICINE*. He saw that most sick people had a digestive system that was running too acidic and gave them simple recipes to become more alkaline. "Over and over, I explain to my patients, Your pain, misery, and illness results from your own dietary mistakes and drugs. You are suffering because you are filled with toxic wastes caused by your diet of poorly selected food filled with artificial flavorings, preservatives, synthetics, and over-processed ingredients-- too much stimulating food and too few natural vitamins from vegetables and fruits..."

"You are what you eat" may not always apply; however, you are what you digest is a likely truism. Point of fact, addressing digestive issues properly can make all the difference for those who have diet fatigue. Studies show that an overgrowth of bad bacteria in the gut can cause inflammation, signaling the fat-regulating hormone leptin to store fat making it difficult to lose weight even when you really try.

The important new field known as Nutrigenomics has demonstrated that approximately one-third of our entire DNA has one simple job: to code for and also produce enzymes controlled by nutrient co-factors. This demonstrates that nutrients have a very powerful ability to modify the expression of our genes. I can only imagine that the opposite may very well be true: that frankenfoods, pesticide residue, and added chemicals can actually alter and damage the expression of our genes.

In the interest of your life long health and happiness as opposed to next summer's bikini body, the following information is critical. I hope that you will use my TWENTY-ONE-DAY CHALLENGE to eliminate your bad habits slowly and take on new habits to heal and nurture yourself, friends, family, and the planet.

1) CLEANSING: I became a veteran faster at twenty after trying the Macrobiotic seven day brown rice regimen. I must really crave discipline because I moved on to juice fasting with the purchase of a Champion juicer and way too many carrots. These seven to ten day bi-annual affairs were complete with colonics and even retention enemas. (A much better way to get your daily Java Boost!) These days, the whole concept of fasting and cleansing has been bumped up a notch by the brilliant work of Jeffry Bland at Metagenics (author of *THE 20-DAY REJUVENATION DIET PROGRAM*). This supplement company has created targeted protein drinks for various metabolic tendencies. Usually, the cleansing begins with a day or two of raw foods which help flush out your system and the program ends with another day or two of raw foods to slowly settle into your lifestyle upgrade. Metagenics is generally available only from Doctors because their supervision is important. Always, when various stressors make me feel vulnerable, it's time to simplify the diet and up the ante on supplements.

2) CONTROL CRAVINGS: If this is your issue, a little psychological leg work can be helpful. For instance, crunchy foods such as salty chips can be very appealing when we're irritated and frustrated, a tough cardio workout may lessen the need. Ditto creamy comfort foods when we need a hug and a friend to listen, sugary foods when we're seeking an afternoon pick-me-up signaling low blood sugar. Joining 'Weight Watchers' or 'Overeaters Anonymous' even for a short time can sharpen your skills here as you will have the benefit of the accumulated experience a group can provide as well as the reckoning where you weigh-in.

3) DIGEST THIS: Believe it or not, digestion begins when we look at our food, smell it and savor the thought of eating it. It gets the juices going... I remind you of this because this step is often entirely skipped with a fast food meal that gets torn open and guzzled down without a glance. Next on the digestive highway is **chewing**, another place where we short change our bodies attempt to function well. Try focusing much more on this process and see what good things might happen. I suggest this be included in your TWENTY-ONE-DAY CHALLENGE, as chewing properly (until the food becomes liquefied) is a form of mindfulness that needs cultivation. (We've grown used to the guzzling!) Cultivating friendly bacteria in our gut is not something many Americans consider other than popping a probiotic pill or downing some sugar laden yogurt but vegans are rediscovering the value of such things as traditionally fermented sauerkraut, Korean Kimchi, and Japanese Miso.

4) EAT BREAKFAST LIKE A KING, lunch like a peasant, and dinner like a pauper. Is there a better way to say pay it forward with food? All of the brilliant metabolic processes that occur as we sleep will occur more brilliantly without the burden of indigestion or heartburn. Of course, for some, breakfast is anathema. For these people as well as those looking for **TRICKS** to help burn more fat: it has been demonstrated that hoping out of bed to exercise immediately for thirty minutes or so will actually target stored fat because there will be no carbohydrates available for fuel. This is not possible for those who have metabolic issues, and a good breakfast is still recommended post exercise. Perhaps by broadening your options for the meal, you can change your mind and consequently shift your metabolism. Personally, I hate orange juice and consider most such beverages to be wasted calories. Far better to eat the fruit and benefit from the fiber. My favorite breakfast at the moment includes a well toasted piece of Food For Life's Brown Rice or Millet Bread topped with a thin shaving of Spanish Manchego Cheese, a tiny slice of avocado, and sometimes a soft boiled egg. Grind Trader Joe's Everyday Seasoning, toss on a few mixed lettuce leaves and voila! Hot tea and a handful of supplements with this combo will keep me going 'til noon.

5) EAT THE RAINBOW: Every week now it seems I am reading about some wonderful new supplement derived from fruits and vegetables. These so called neutraceuticals are readily available in the original sources for a fraction of the cost of the supplement and they are a wonderful investment in your health. Personally, I strive to consume five to ten different and brightly colored fruits and vegetables each day. My energy and mood is always greatly enhanced when I make the effort. On a busy day when I know it can't happen, I might order a fresh large mixed veggie juice at Whole Foods or the CO-OP. Instant energy, calm nerves, glowing skin, what's not to like? If I'm feeling low, I might add a big wallop of fresh ginger and garlic…. If you want to target your consumption of fruits and vegetables to heal specific conditions, I recommend a book called *NATURE'S RECIPE FOR PEAK HEALTH*. This "Antidote for Commercialized Medicine" is both helpful and fascinating.

6) ELIMINATE SODAS: Most people like to think diet soda is better. Is it? I gave it up and I'll tell you why: First of all, it's a chemical cocktail (unless you buy organic and sugar free) and secondly, it triggers a thirst for more sweet tastes, it keeps the sugar addiction going. Often, it keeps the caffeine addiction going as well-

7) ELIMINATE THE WHITES: I am not talking about the very occasional slice of celebratory cake or shared desert after a fine dining experience. I am talking about how you start your day and how you fuel your body. It is what we do each day habitually that creates our health or it's absence. These white refined products are at the top of the glycemic index charts because regular consumption is so detrimental. Not only are you not getting the fuel you need to run a mean machine, but, if we had a similar grade school experience, you may recall making paste with white flour and water... thinking, huh? Whole grains are everywhere now (what with excessive pretty packaging, too); you have no excuses for failing to experiment!

8) DIETS THAT WORK: Lot's of popular and workable diets have featured the balance of proteins, fats, and carbs and are generally a variation of the classic Mediterranean diet. Years ago, I tried the Atkins diet for a week and it made me feel nauseous. The newer version, the Paleo diet appears to be much healthier for long term living. I tried Macrobiotics as well as vegetarianism in my youth and they made me feel sluggish. These days, I consider myself to be flexitarian in that I consume an abundance of fresh fruits and vegetables whenever possible, preferably organic. (For a farmer's market near you, check www.localharvest.org.) If I can add wild caught fish and free range chicken, turkey, or eggs once or twice a week, great. Otherwise, I make myself a smoothie. I might use a whey protein powder or soak raw almonds, rub the skin off and toss them into the blender with papaya, mango or pineapple, banana, berries (any of these can be frozen) and sometimes a few leafy greens. I admit that I am quite enthralled with the current offerings of prepared raw foods for vegans, I've had some divine kale chips and truly heavenly chocolate deserts that did not spike my blood sugar I still love pastries: whole grain, organic, and very rarely. I too have the dread 'diabesity' genes lurking inside and I begin salivating as I write about chocolate and pastry!

9) FOOD INTOLERANCE: eating foods that are not compatible with your bodies biochemistry can cause cellular inflammation and insulin resistance, causing them to be stored as fat instead of being burned. The ALCAT test is now readily available to determine food and chemical sensitivities. While many have adopted a gluten free diet in hopes of eliminating allergens, precisely pinpointing your sensitivities has been very helpful to many. Additionally, a 'gluten free' diet may help you lose weight simply because it can cause you to cut down on your intake of carbohydrates from grains- if this is your goal, be wary of all the baked goods on the market now catering to the needs of individuals with Celiac disease as sugar and many other possible irritants are often prominently featured in these items.

10) GET GOOD SALT: In Finland, a nationwide use of a reduced sodium formula implemented in nineteen ninety-six resulted in a sixty percent decrease in deaths from stroke and heart disease. Dr. Jonathan Wright sells this formula on his Tahoma Clinic Dispensary website. I've long been a fan of the French formula called 'Herbamare' and most recently, I am impressed with Trader Joe's 'Everyday Seasoning' which comes in a grinder. "Nature's Recipe For Peak Health" (see # II above) also includes specialty salt recipes for those who like to do it yourself.

11) PREPARATION METHODS: most of us are aware by now that over cooking destroys many valuable nutrients in fruits and vegetables. However, you may be unaware that the microwave, while it may actually enhance certain vitamins in vegetables, is detrimental to the amino acid chains in meats and may impair their digestibility. (I just did a fact check on this and it was frightening!) Also, if you are a fan of the barbecue, keep in mind that the crusty black 'char' is actually highly carcinogenic. It can be reduced by keeping the grill clean of these particles and by using a marinade that features olive oil with a little lemon juice and the addition of herbs such as rosemary, thyme, sage, oregano, basil, or mint. Also, this may be old news, but the non-stick pan may not be so wonderful. Ditto with aluminum pans....

12) PURE WATER: This is a critical component for your health and fitness lifestyle. I purchased a small WATERWISE distiller and I couldn't be happier. For years I had distilled water delivered in five gallon bottles but the company decided to stop using glass bottles. Since I mentioned bottling, beware of always drinking from plastic bottles, even if the bottles are Bp free, there is probably leakage of other chemicals into the water. If you have concerns that you will be lacking minerals, you can add some liquid minerals to the water. Distilled water makes the most delicious teas and coffees. This will save you big bucks over time!

13) READ LABELS: We are very lucky to have all the pertinent information on our labels these days. While the latest research indicates that it may not be as simple (or ineffective for some!) as calories in verses calories burned, common sense suggests that figuring the number of calories required to maintain your ideal body weight will at least be a helpful measure of portion size. If you stick to an active lifestyle, you may be able to burn a few more as I understand there is something called a 'window of opportunity' which occurs after an intense aerobic activity... all careers have their little perks! While I'm on the subject of labels and perks- go to www.foodnews.org for your free wallet sized downloadable card that lists the dirty dozen foods that you should avoid unless you find certified organic as well as the consistently clean which are better purchased from a local source.

EXTREME REMEDIES

"Try and fail, but don't fail to try."
~ Stephen Kaggwa

"The Devil has put a penalty on all things we enjoy in life.
Either we suffer in health or we suffer in soul or we get fat."
~ Albert Einstein

"She must have been very strictly brought up,
she's so desperately anxious to do
the wrong thing correctly."
~ H. H. Munro

Susan Uppington-Smyth has been taking my "Making Waves" class for many months now and it seems that everyone at the gym has been following her story with interest. Susan recently had bariatric bypass surgery and has literally, in her own words, "lost her Mother", (that's one hundred-forty pounds to date, and still losing). Some of you who purchase this book may know Susan, and know that we have changed her name in these pages. Susan is successfully using every means at her disposal to reinvent herself as a healthier, happier person. It cannot be easy, mid journey, to share her history and I am most grateful to her, as I know the retelling had to bring up lots of old feelings...

"My story is not that exciting. I was not abused in any sort of way. I have not had any major tragedies, no hardships. In fact, I had a very good life. My parents loved me and gave me every advantage they could (except for the horse I wanted, but in hindsight that was a good thing, horses scare me). The friends that I made in childhood are still my friends today. I excelled academically during my school years. However, from day one I was, as my Daddy put it, on the opposite ends of the height-weight chart (and not the tall/ thin way)."

"I am not saying that my life was perfect, it wasn't. It had its ups and downs, but in all honesty, nothing that was out of the ordinary. My parents were extremely strict and I very much wanted to please them. I always did what I was told. However, I was a very literal person. When I was told something, I took it to heart and kept it there for a very long time, especially when I made mistakes. I had a difficult time recovering from my mistakes and disappointments. I over thought these things and refused to let them go. I just added them to an ever-increasing list of what is wrong with me, which wreaked havoc with my self-confidence and my self-esteem."

"I was an extremely 'good girl'. I didn't rebel, except with food. Food was the only thing I could control. I would use food for every emotion: lonely, upset, heartbroken, sad, happy, excited, tired."

"As a pre-teen, I tried everything from Weight Watchers to joining a magic mirror salon. In case you don't remember what a magic mirror salon was, it was one of those old fashioned women's gyms, with the vibrating belts and other equipment you see on old I LOVE LUCY reruns. I even tried

Dexitrim when I was twelve years old! That only happened once, because I spent the rest of the day shaking, crying, and listening to Queen's THE GAME album."

"Even at that young age, I had countless books on the subject of dieting. One book that stands out in my mind was targeted toward teenage girls. At the time, it was probably the only diet book for girls. My memories of this bright pink hardback book are quite specific, though I am not certain they are accurate. The diet specified in those pages was quite unremarkable and typical for that time-- grapefruit and cottage cheese. The remainder of the book consisted of such information as how to keep your hair nice and wear nice clothes. For some reason, this made me really mad. Not only was I fat, I was being told that I was unkempt. Another item to add to my list of mistakes. Of course, these diets did not work for me because I did not want to diet and was angry that I needed to. My food was a necessary coping mechanism."

"In high school, I decided that I wanted to go to boarding school for my junior and senior years. (I actually wanted to go and I loved it!) So, I got my freshmen fifteen (or thirty) done a couple of years early and in high school. Although I was no longer under the watchful eyes of my parents, I was still a 'good girl' and did what I was told, while continuing to use food to medicate my emotions. At boarding school, I didn't have the same pressures I had experienced in public school. I was not expected to make straight A's. I did just fine academically, but I no longer had a 4.0 grade point average. My parents were happy with my grades, but a part of me was disappointed in myself. The tapes that I played in my head still said that I had to be perfect to please my parents."

"I went on to college and continued to steadily gain a few more pounds each year. The next stop for me on the diet train was the liquid diet. Oprah Winfrey had just had incredible success with the liquid diet and so I was quick to try it also. That was not the diet program for me. The protein shakes made my stomach get so upset. At one point, I had to drink them in a bathroom stall because I was so close to throwing up. After that attempt, I tried the cookie diet, followed by Nutrisystem."

"During my last year of college my father died. Although he had been sick for a year, it was still more upsetting for me than expected. I was quite devastated. I was a daddy's girl. My father was the one who comforted me. He was an extremely kind and ethical man. I missed him terribly then and I still do today. Feeling very fragile, I was not ready for the uncertainty of the real world, so I opted for grad school."

"Not surprisingly, my rate of weight gain escalated. I finished grad school and moved to the west coast to work. I landed my dream job and worked my way up through the ranks. Just like life, the job had its ups and downs. My desire to please my parents transferred to my desire to please my boss. I obsessed about losing my job and I coped with that emotion by eating. I gained ten to twenty pounds a year for the next fifteen years. Every mistake I made went on my list and to this day, those mistakes still cause me anxiety. Food once again was my coping tool."

"During these years, I still tried more diets like South Beach and Atkins. I even tried Nutrisystem two more times, along with dietitians and therapy. Twice, I lost forty pounds, and then gained it back. Once with Weight Watchers and then another medically supervised fast. It is very hard to stay with a plan when you don't like the food or the meal replacement shakes. You would think by now I would have learned that these plans don't work for me long term."

"At this point, I decided that I needed to have the surgery. This was not an easy decision. I really did not want to go that route. I had heard for so many years about the problems that people had after the surgery. But after four different doctors suggested that I have it, I began investigating the possibility for myself. With the first weight loss surgery program, I was told to come back after I lost five percent of my body weight and they would then schedule me for the surgery. When I was unable to accomplish this in the designated time frame, the program coordinator yelled at me for wasting time. Clearly, this was not the program for me."

"Although I was still working at my dream job, the environment had turned toxic. I would on most days, eat only once. I would get to the office early, work through lunch and have a large meal delivered to me at night. My go to food was fried cheese, coke, and a hamburger or pizza. I would come home from work and be so hungry, that I felt I'd go crazy if I didn't have fried cheese very soon."

"Then, after more than fifteen years with the same company, I lost my job. Again, I was devastated and my self-confidence hit rock bottom. But, like the old Rolling Stones song goes, 'You can't always get what you want, but if you try sometimes, you just might find, you get what you need'. Being out of work gave me the opportunity to get serious about my weight problem. After several months of depression and the addition of forty more pounds, I was finally able to commit to losing the weight that was required of me before surgery and finding the right program for me. Because I am an emotional eater, the stressors at work were making it impossible for me to lose weight. I had been completely unable to breakaway from the life long habits I'd relied upon to cope with the pressures of the work place environment."

THE PROCESS

"Once I was in the right program for me, it took about nine months from start to surgery. Notice I didn't say from start to finish, because I will never be finished. The surgery that rearranged my insides will force me to be very aware of what I am eating for the rest of my life."

"Before I was able to have the appointment with the doctor, I had to attend the hospital's introductory seminar. The seminar included an overview of the different types of weight loss surgery and what to expect from the surgery and afterwards as well."

"The staff was very organized and had scheduled the appointment with the surgeon for later that same day. I met with the doctor and we decided the best surgery for me would be gastric bypass and we discussed what my next steps would be. Since I was so huge, he also required me to lose some weight and sent me to the risk reduction doctor. Here, I was put on a diet of shakes and meal replacements. I also began a mandatory nutrition class on a weekly basis. Oh no, not again!"

"The shakes were slightly better than the ones I'd had earlier and the meal replacements were pre-portioned shelf stable meals that were ok. But of course, I could not make it easy. I had a terrible time tolerating the shakes and I am such a picky eater that I would only eat two or three of the varieties of meal replacements. So, that was not really working for me. Fortunately, the nutrition class gave me the skills to let me eat conventional foods and still lose the weight."

"Finally, I learned that instead of budgeting a daily calorie limit, **(TIP) I could count calories on a weekly basis**. This gave me the opportunity to enjoy eating things that I really liked as long as I could work them into my calorie budget. Looking at it from a weekly perspective kept me from experiencing the crushing defeat that made it really hard to start the diet over again the next day. In addition, with all the new technology, tracking the calories became so much easier. I no longer had to carry around calorie books and note books to track my meals, preplanning was now much easier. I was able to log on to the computer or phone and record my calories."

"The program also required me to meet one on one with a psychologist and a dietitian. The psychologist was to make sure I was able to comply with the doctor's orders. The dietitian went over the various supplements that I will have to take for the rest of my life as well as what I would be able to eat post surgery."

"As I got closer to my targeted weight and the surgery itself, I had a few pre-op procedures. The first test was an EDG (esophagogastroduodenoscopy), where they put you out for a few minutes to stick a camera down your throat and make sure your stomach is ok. The second test was a cardiac stress test. Because of my size, I was not able to use a treadmill, so the doctors used drugs to make my heart race. If I had a gall bladder, I would have also had an abdominal ultrasound."

"After six months of the nutrition classes, I had lost forty pounds and my risk reduction doctor approved me for surgery. The next step was to submit the paperwork to my bariatric caseworker and wait to get approval from the insurance company. Here, I was extremely lucky! I was approved and given a surgery date within two hours of the submission. DON'T EXPECT THAT TO HAPPEN."

"My surgery date was in three weeks. For the two weeks prior to the surgery, I was on a very strict diet of mostly liquids and one meal per day. The reason for this, besides the extra weight loss, was to shrink the liver and give the surgeon more room to work in the abdomen. Two days before surgery, I went on clear liquids only in order to clear out the digestive tract."

"I don't remember much about the surgery or the hospital recovery, however, it is very important to follow your doctors orders. Basically, you need to get in your fluids and your protein. Also, you must get up and walk around."

"Once I was back home, I began my prescribed **Diet Progression**. If you elect this surgical procedure, it is essential that you follow your doctor's orders, which may differ, from mine:

Week **1):** Clear liquids and Protein Supplements
Week **2):** Full liquids and Protein Supplements
(and pureed non- cream soups)

Week **3 and 4):** Pureed and Mashed Foods
Week **5):** Chopped foods
Week **6):** Solid foods

In addition to the diet progression, here are a few of the many **Rules**, which you must follow:

1): Don't drink for thirty minutes after your meal, it could flush the food out of your pouch too fast.
2): Eat your protein first.
3): Take thirty minutes to eat a meal.
4): Drink your required amount of fluids.
5): Meet your protein goals.
6): Stop if you are full.

One reason I chose the surgery is that I am pretty good at following rules, when I have to. During my pre-surgery weight loss, I was able to work some of my favorite/ trigger foods (fried cheese and coke) into my calorie budget. More specifically, I still had the choice to eat those foods. After surgery, those choices were taken away. I can't have fried foods (good bye fried cheese!) or carbonated beverages (so long coke, my old friend). And to be perfectly honest, it hasn't really been a problem to cut those things out since these kinds of foods now present very real medical consequences for me."

"The surgery is just a tool, it is not a magic fix-all. I have to spend more time thinking and planning my food than I ever did pre-surgery. I can no longer eat whatever I want, whenever I want. I have to get up every morning and make sure I have all my food planned out, so I meet my protein and calorie goals. "

"For me, the surgery took away the ability to use my trigger foods as a coping mechanism. I have to find another way to cope."

"If you are considering weight loss surgery, do your research. Find a good program and a good experienced surgeon. "

"The following **TIPS** are a few things I wish I had known from the start. It would have saved me a lot of time and grief:

1) Contact your **Insurance** company first thing. If weight loss surgery is covered, they may require participation in a medically supervised/documented program before they will grant approval. In my opinion, there is no downside to doing this immediately. Even if you decide not to have the surgery; you will still have started on your weight loss journey. You may, in fact, find that you can lose the weight without the surgery.

2) Find the right **Program/Hospital** for you. My first program was not comprehensive. I was told to lose five percent of my body weight and given a set of dietary guidelines. *If I could lose weight doing that, I wouldn't need surgery!* In addition, the program coordinator was verbally abusive to me several times. Sadly, this was a world-renowned hospital! Fortunately, I discovered another program that was organized and had all aspects covered. They administered a weight loss class that helped me pass insurance approval and no one ever yelled at me.

3) Vitamins are mandatory post surgery and I should have known from my previous experience that they would present a challenge. I would become nauseated after taking them for a couple days. In retrospect, I should have taken them for a substantial period of time before the surgery to make sure I could tolerate them afterwards.

4) Time Management post surgery is very intensive. Previously, I would eat one meal a day and now, I must eat four to five small meals daily plus they require coordination with my vitamin and fluid schedule.

5) I highly recommend **www.myfitnesspal.com**. You can link my 'fitbit' (www.fitbit.com) which tracks your steps, stairs climbed, calories burned... it can even track your sleep! The neat thing is, you can link myfitnesspal with fitbit (www.myfitnesspal.com/apps/show/fitbit) so that our food can be factored in.

6) Recently, I've discovered a fun set of tools and great information at **www.lifesizeportions.com.** They can help you find ways to eat a little extra food in a meal without eating too many extra calories.

Weight loss surgery is just a tool. I still have to do the work and it is a lot of work. At this point, I am a little over three months out of surgery and have lost one hundred pounds (including my pre-surgery weight loss). I still have a very long way to go. My weight loss has been consistent but slow.

Water exercise, has been a lifesaver for me because I wasn't able to expend much energy with land based exercise. At my size, I was afraid I would break the equipment in the gym or worse, that it might break me. I really didn't want to go to the doctor to hear "I can't help you because of your weight." (Yes, that really happened when I twisted my knee!) This past summer, there has been a marked increase in the duration and intensity of my performance. I do my morning class with Janna, then return home for lunch and another hour in the pool at home. Some weeks, I did as much as nine hours in the pool.

With my weight loss, my range of motion has increased and I am finally able to perform some of the yoga poses that are done at the end of class. I can now grab my foot in the runner's stretch and grasp my hands behind my back. (This makes me very happy because I can now scratch much more of my back!) I was able to share a laugh with my friends at Janna's "Making Waves" aquatic exercise class last week. After the prior days class, I was on the elevator heading home, when I looked down at the floor and, much to my surprise, I saw a big pool of my black granny panties. Fortunately, the skirt I was wearing, while hanging low, was keeping me covered. Thank goodness I was alone and happened to know that the surveillance camera didn't work. I wouldn't want that on the Internet! I'm feeling pretty good about myself these days. For me, surgery was the best decision and I am happy I did it."

SUPPLEMENT THIS!

"If it came in a bottle,
everybody would have a great body"
~ Cher

"There are no facts, only interpretations."
~ Friedrich Nietzsche

"A man's health can be judged by that
which he takes two at a time-pills or stairs."
~ Joan Welsh

I just got off the phone with my new friend Lesly. We were both guests at a lovely Memorial Day party in historic Beachwood Canyon where we sipped Mojitos beneath the famous 'Hollywood' sign. She'd heard our mutual friends commenting about how busy I've been, working on this book and training. "You must be teaching how many classes per week?" She'd enquired that day. "Twelve or so", I replied,"then there's the occasional private". "How do you do it?" Lesly asked. "Well, I love me some DHEA!" I responded, feeling silly 'cause I'm such a cheap drunk (as are most athletic people with a healthy liver). But yes, I do love me some DHEA and I thank my lucky stars that it's legal- otherwise; I could be tempted to a life of crime!

Now, I've got Lesly on the phone wanting to know "What exactly does it do? Can I take it too?" Well, I'm not a doctor and I don't pretend to know if it's really a good thing for Lesly. She's a beautiful post-menopausal brunette using a patch and some other prescriptions from her gynecologist. We talked about it ... how she could easily try a little and see how ten milligrams feels for her. But, I cautioned her; it's used usually in conjunction with Pregnenalone to help balance your hormones. If you're already taking something with hormones, even that little bit might throw your whole system out of kilter.

Lesly is doing the smart thing and calling her GYN. She's also doing the inspired thing and ordering up one of Suzanne Summer's books at Amazon.com. Oh, for a piece of the action on book sales for S.S's! Let me say right here and now what I wish someone could have said to me at the age of thirty-five, go get tested soon when you are at your peak of health and vitality. You will want a full panel of hormone testing so that you have the option to replicate this precious balance later on when your system starts to fail you.

There are some brilliant Doctors (most listed in S.S's. books) who can look you over and make a well educated guess about your needs. Those of us who missed the boat on prime time blood testing are lucky to work with these guys. However, it isn't inexpensive and not necessarily covered by insurance, another reason to invest in testing at thirty-five! With these tests, you won't have to have a brilliant Doctor ... one that you like and trust will do. If you're one of those naturalists determined to accept dwindling hormones as a normal phenomenon with age, I highly recommend that you make provisions for a possible change of mind when you actually get 'the change of life'.

While you're at it, you might consider banking your own DNA as insurance against a host of diseases that may be part of your inherited genetic predisposition. You'll have to budget it carefully as it's akin to purchasing a nice used car in today's market but that is nothing compared to the added years of health and happiness it might provide down the road.

Least I forget, I don't mean to leave you hanging with questions about DHEA, since I praised it for my own use. Pharma-phobe that I generally am, I do sing its praises, but let me caution you with the information on the label:

'Not for use by individuals under the age of eighteen years. Do not use if pregnant or nursing. Consult a physician or other licensed qualified health care professional before using this product if you have or have a family history of, prostate cancer, prostate enlargement, heart disease, low "good" cholesterol (HDL), or if you are using any other dietary supplement, prescription drug, or over-the-counter drug. Do not exceed recommended serving. Exceeding recommended serving may cause aggressiveness, irritability, and increased levels of estrogen. Discontinue use and call physician immediately if you experience rapid heartbeat, dizziness, blurred vision, or other similar symptoms.'

Nice huh! New information presents itself all the time and I recently read that a sub-lingual delivery system such as drops or spray is best... but seldom available, in my experience. I admit, I did over-do-it a few years ago, shortly after discovering it. But that's because most of the literature pushes twenty-five to fifty milligrams and that became too much for me. When I found myself overcome by road rage, I decided to cut back to ten mg. A well informed clerk in my favorite discount vitamin store inquired whether I realized it was better to take it with Pregnenalone for a woman my age (it comes together in some capsules) and I bless him for insisting that I should take DIM (a compound found in cruciferous vegetables like broccoli and cauliflower) as well, to help protect against cancer.

Sorry to be a little boring with this tale but I think it represents the dilemma we face when discovering and implementing new information about supplements as well as diet and exercise. We live in the information age and the info keeps coming and sometimes it seems to (outright!) contradict what we thought they knew already... I admit I am my own guinea pig but I take full responsibility for my well-being. After all, if I cared absolutely about my health as a first priority, I would move away from LA. As it is, I trained as an instructor of applied Kinesiology and simple muscle testing can be a useful tool to test for efficacy of many vitamins and allergens as well.

I do firmly believe that most of us city dwellers are suffering from what's been termed 'Nature Deficit Disorder' (to quote author Richard Louv) and it makes sense when you consider that our environment is polluted and even our freshest food tends to be way old before it gets consumed. Not to mention the fact that it's packaged, processed, and frequently grown with shelf life as a priority.

If you can treat yourself to a good nutritionist, you may get the help you need in making some smart and affordable choices for supplementation. If dollars are tight right now, take advantage of on-line research to determine what you must have if you want to thrive and not just survive. Then, there's always the clerk at the vitamin store, if you find one who has a real interest in his work, he can, indeed, be a blessing to you...

Before moving on here, I want to give you a few **TIPS** that apply to the questions my friends and clients most frequently ask, though I reference these here in hopes that you will discuss them in consultation with a professional:

1) A Supplement Break - Since we are all creatures of habit who seem to adapt to whatever we do regularly, I find it useful (as well as economical) to take a break (at least annually, or when I run out) from my regular regimen. I prefer to do this in the summer with a cleansing program that includes green juices, fresh vegetables and fruits. However, an after-the-Holiday's cleanse that features a rich hot potassium broth (organic potato peels with just enough potato meal to thicken the broth), green beans, zucchini, curry spices such as turmeric and ginger, garlic, etc., can be both a fresh start on the new year and a hedge against January colds and flu.

2) Be Right with the B's - The B's are a no brainer because we urinate and they disappear down the tank in a bright yellow swirl. It's an insufficient quantity in the tired foods we consume that plague us in the city... If you are vegetarian or vegan, you might need B12 supplementation as deficiencies may lead to loss of vision, delusional behavior, sadness, depression, or even personality changes as well as developmental delays in children. Also, in any wellness program, it helps to remember that the B's boost detoxification. If you have a stressful life style, it's safe to say "take your B complex"!

3) Colds and Flu : Dr. Mark Hyman just offered some very useful info in his news letter about Flu shots. If you choose to get one, he suggests the mercury-free (Thimerosal is a preservative) version. Choosing a single dose or pre-filled syringe can give you that option. As for me, I'm quite 'old school' in this regard. I seldom get sick, but when I do, it's usually only three days. I figure the germs are everywhere but it's my resistance that's down. Bed rest, chicken soup or a veggie mineral rich broth (organic potato skins, carrots for beta-carotene, etc.) and the natural anti-viral mediterranean oil of oregano as well as colloidal silver spray and goldenseal capsules can do wonders. So many people pop an antibiotic right away, wiping out all the friendly bacteria in their system and possibly building resistance to antibiotics. As for the confusion over that old saying "feed a cold, starve a fever", science seems to support the idea that 'catching a chill' may be responsible in colds and nourishment may be helpful, while the tendency to fever with flu is better dealt with by consuming plenty of fluids.

4) Conflicting Information - How much vitamin "D" is right for you? Do you really need massive doses of calcium? (This is big as of this writing because some studies have shown an increase in heart attacks and kidney stones with excessive supplementation; unlike eating calcium rich foods.) Is magnesium equally or even more important to your body type? Are you able to assimilate what you take? Be wary of mega doses and approach all new information conservatively, else you may, at the least, be wasting big bucks and putting yourself at risk. I did a series of colonics some years ago and my knowledgeable practitioner was kind enough to point out all the undigested huge tablets I had been consuming. Now,

I stick to gelatin capsules and gel formulas. I generally prefer to take quality supplements individually or bunched together as in the B's and a mineral complex. A multi-vitamin/ mineral supplement from a reputable company can be very helpful if your diet is inconsistent, but I would *never expect it to be a replacement for eating well* on a regular basis.

5) Digestive Aids - Toxic build up in the gut is responsible for killing off the healthy flora as is antibiotic use and acute stress which results in bloat and inflammation that can signal the fat-regulating hormone leptin to store fat. Since fixing your gut can result in losing it, the results of a targeted cleanse can be life changing. If your Doctor agrees, a couple weeks on an herbal antimicrobial formula such as Allergy Research Group's Tricycline combined with a cleansing diet that eliminates caffeine, alcohol, sugar, gluten, processed foods, and dairy (even yogurt), as well as sugar dense fruits and the higher glycemic vegetables should eliminate the bad bacteria. A digestive enzyme supplement such as BodHD's BLB taken during this process will give your system a boost. The next two weeks supplement with the amino-acid L-glutamine to help heal the gut wall and add a probiotic to replace healthy bacteria. Some consider the probiotic to be the single most important thing you can do to improve digestion, decrease inflammation, and boost immunity. If this sounds like a daunting ordeal, try loosely following the diet and taking the probiotic, it just might do the **TRICK** for improved digestion and a flater tummy.

6) Fat Burning Aids - If you're looking for a quick education on supplements that aid this process, go to www.bodybuilding.com and check out all the latest products on the market as well as dietary tips. Beware of trendy items such as Raspberry Ketones, the most recent buzz in the fat burning world along with green coffee. It seems the quality product may have some usefulness, but unfortunately, the synthesized versions, and/ or cheap versions appear soon after and you may be wasting your dollars on junk. If your weight issues are about stubborn middle-aged belly fat, consider Dr. Steven Sisskind's "Real Dose" weight loss formula available at Amazon. His online video about the superior ingredients is very convincing. Also, I would check out www.thyrophoenix.com as it is a terrific resource for helping to determine (as I have) whether the addition of a daily drop of inexpensive liquid potassium iodide might rev up your metabolism, help protect against breast cancer and excessive radiation exposure. Other simple and inexpensive **TRICKS** include developing a taste for 'hot' cayenne chili seasonings as well as green tea and even drinking cold water which can cause you to burn a few more calories ... If you can hop out of bed in the morning and do 10 - 30 minutes of exercise, especially intense aerobic activity, the new thinking is it burns stored fat because there is no other fuel available until after you eat.

7) Hair Loss in Women - I don't know whether this problem has become more pronounced or whether there are just more of us getting older but clients continually ask me to tell them what I know... (Some causes are stress and/ or age related related and estrogen deficiency related as testosterone can become more dominate.) Right now, there is in Hollywood a run on 'Viviscal', which is a Marine Complex capsule. I am testing it now, four months into it and thinking my hair may be slightly fluffier. I will persist, as we all want it to work! I have also increased my biotin consumption to a greater degree than what was in my B-complex capsule. Another choice available online and offering a money back guarantee is Hair Essentials. I am already taking many of the items in this product, so read the label! Shampoo's and treatment products that may help **Men and Women** include the famous Nioxin line for aging or thinning hair as well as an upscale version of the old apple cider vinegar rinse (supposedly, it dissolves that nasty DHT build up in the hair follicles) available at www.justnaturalskincare.com. The latest research cited in the *THE WALL STREET JOURNAL* suggests we may soon be reawakening sleeping hair follicles by targeting vitamin D receptors and/ or growing stem cells and and turning them into hair producing follicles.

8) Joint Integrity - Supplementation that addresses these issues can become expensive- Glucosamine and Chondroitin have been positively reviewed though many people fail to take the necessary amount for their body weight and fail to take it consistently for three to six months. In doing a little additional research, I see that some Chiropractors feel that 1500 mg daily of Glucosamine coupled with 2-3000 mg of MSM is a better way to go as they cite low efficacy of Chondroitin because it's chemical structure is so large. Hyaluronic Acid can be helpful with cushioning the joints as well as maintaining the elastic integrity of skin.

9) Longevity - we are beginning to understand that a continuing youthful expression of our genes as well as Telomere length (the protective tip) on the strands of DNA is very influenced by what we ingest. Slowing the aging process appears to be aided by Omega 3 Fatty Acids with EPA and DHA, Resveratrol, Vitamins A,B,C,D,E, Alpha Lipoic Acid,and Carnosine. A new supplement called TA-65 is supposedly most efficacious but appears to rival the fabled Chinese Ginseng when it comes to cost. And speaking of price points, a good anti-aging doctor is a necessity if you're going to track your physical response to a supplement regime that often recommends mega-doses. This could get expensive! it might be wise not to discuss with children who might fear their inheritance could go up in smoke...

10) Mood Stabilization - you may be rather young but plagued by symptoms that you or your well meaning Doctor treat with antidepressant medication. Are we not the Prozac Nation? Realizing you are not meant to stay on antidepressants indefinitely, be smart and read up (www.amenclinics.com). Sometimes all that may be required is a supervised regime to address exhausted adrenal glands and/ or hormone imbalance. After some weeks of treatment, you may be able to transition to a 'natural' formula (such as Stress Factors by Biogenesis) that can help support mood stabilization. I know I had some very dark days in my teens and it always seemed a cosmic joke when 'Flo" showed up a day or two later. Getting off of sugar, burgers, and fries can make all the difference in the world, in addition to regular exercise. It takes a little time to transition away from a pharmaceutical fix (and perhaps not everyone can) but your future health depends on it as the latest studies confirm.

11) Muscle Building Aids - I refer you again to www.bodybuilding.com. Both the prices and the products are impressive. Information, motivation, and supplementation are at your finger tips along with tools to track your progress. There are many good deals on whey protein which is a useful and easy to use staple of the now classic 'smoothie' meal replacement for those on the go. I like to keep frozen mango, banana, berries, and pineapple on hand as well as fresh papaya, a tasty combo with a good vanilla whey. My favorite mix master at Whole Foods would like to make a chocolate version with sprouted organic oats and almonds. If you need an added sweet taste, try liquid or powdered stevia.

12) Phytonutrients Rule! - Everyday, it seems they are discovering some new miracle compound in spices, herbs, wine, dark chocolate, brightly colored fruits, veggies, even tree bark, algae and many more. I could go 'hog wild' on these things but for the expense and perhaps it's just as well that my emphasis be on *consuming the actual food*. However, if, for instance, you suspect Alzheimer's lurks in your future, why not consider a quality brand and high concentration of Resveratrol? Ditto for Curcumin, the potent substance derived from turmeric which is being studied for it's effect on tumors and cancer. In India, where the bright, yellow orange root is a classic ingredient in curries, the incidence of Alzheimer's is one-sixth that of the United States.

13) Sugar addiction - My old favorite, Dr. Henry Bieler wrote about addiction and how many recovering addicts get off of booze and take up a sugar addiction in it's place. He suggested that the stomach becomes a distillery... The latest research demonstrates that there is an ineffective dopamine reward response causing addicts to need extra stimulation to turn on the pleasure gene. The Amino Acids Glutamine, Tyrosine, and 5-HTP may help reduce cravings as can sufficient Vitamin D. If this is a serious issue for you, please check out www.dr.hyman.com. If the word 'Diabesity' speaks to you, he's your man. I recommend you get on his e-mail list as it's always great information from an expert. Additionally, I like the www.tahomaclinic blog where you can read about berberine and cinnamon.

14) Sun Protection - If you'r fair skinned and anxious about being in the outdoors because screen doesn't quite do it for you, consider supplements featuring Polypodium Leucotomas,an extract from ferns available in Heliocare and similar preparations. The online Tahoma Clinic Pharmacy offers Dr. Jonathan Wright's preparation which features a full array of supplementation factors for sun exposure protection.

15) Supplementing Hormones - All of the best doctors who give interviews are in agreement that even bioidentical hormones must be balanced. I discussed this at the opening of this chapter but feel it merits further consideration. Ask your health care provider about a twenty-four hour urine test. If you begin a program with your physician, you will want to track those numbers as your hormonal balance improves. I am talking to you *guys* here too!

16) The Omega Dilemma - Do you regularly consume fish such a wild salmon? How about fresh nuts, seeds and their butters? If not, consider supplementation. Evening Primrose oil, Flax oil, Borage, as well as fish oils and special combinations of all the above can do wonders for your fitness and beauty (not to mention your heart and brain!).

17) Vitamin C Calibration - Here is a real life saver... I know because it saved mine! In a pinch, I would try any good crystalline "C" for this procedure but my sister turned me on to this when I suffered a horrible allergy rash-inflammation at Christmas two years ago. I didn't know if it was Holiday travel induced stress or food allergies. (I was losing weight because everything seemed to make it worse!) My sister's husband is a Gastroenterologist but it is Linda who studies her supplements. Her brilliant product, "Perque Potent C

Guard" offers detailed instructions for a "calibration" where you take a spoonful in a glass of good water every 15 minutes until you feel like you're gonna explode. You get the runs but that's nothing when you wake up the next morning with glowing rash free skin. Of course, there are many symptoms of *inflammation* besides rashes that can benefit from this recalibration and it will help you establish the dosage which will be of maximum benefit.

A BRAINSTORM

"I have to exercise in the morning
before my brain figures out what I'm doing."

~ Marsha Doble

"Education is a progressive discovery of our own ignorance."
~ Will Durant

"The brain is a wonderful organ; it starts working the moment you get up in the morning and does not stop until you get into the office."
~ Robert Frost

"The difference between genius
and stupidity is that genius has its limits."
~ Albert Einstein

I've just exhausted myself looking at videos on YouTube about Karl Pribram and his major life's work on the brain as a Hologram. This concept has always been intriguing to me as it explains so many things while simultaneously opening our minds to vast possibilities... Karl states "the world of appearances (what we see through the lens of our eye) is flat while the world at a greater distance is round". We remember that Pythagoras first postulated this in five hundred seventy

BC but it wasn't 'til we traveled the globe that it gained traction. Now that we can observe the Earth spinning about it's orbit from space, we laugh at the ignorance of those who believed the world was flat.

In the coming paradigm shift, science will tackle problems that have been left to the nonscientists; to parapsychologists, to mystics. A Biblical statement such as "You are in the image of God..." is a holographic-like statement that Karl explores to demonstrate the merging of scientific research and mysticism. Some of you readers may well remember the release of the book *WHY GOD WON'T GO AWAY* by Andrew Newberg which galvanized our attention with SPECT scanning showing the actual neural activity in brains that were experiencing intense spiritual peaks.

I've lost two friends to brain tumors in recent years and both of them drove home this idea of the brain as a hologram. My female friend had had the state of the art surgery claiming that her brain was in the Smithsonian Museum. Blindness was a consequence, which prompted the sad necessity of having to go home to live with her eighty-year-old mom. Other than that, her good humor and mental agility were an inspiration to all. My male friend, on the other hand, I suspect (retrospectively) knew this might be his genetic destiny as a brain tumor had killed his own mother at forty-nine. His lifestyle and diet were among the healthiest of all the people I've ever known, so friends were shocked when he was found incoherently walking the streets of New York City. What was more shocking was the way he shunned medical intervention; claiming, "this will all be over in two weeks". Which it was... precisely!

This is all quite fascinating stuff and useful to ponder in light of the ignorance we have regarding neurodegenerative disorders such as Alzheimer's and Parkinson's disease. Current research suggests that while these conditions can have many different triggers, they might act through a common mechanism to damage nerve cells. Recent UK research presents the appealing concept that one treatment; a protein injection, may be useful in stopping degeneration and restoring normal function in all neurodegenerative disease.

Surveys indicate that forty-five percent of Americans mistakenly believe that there is a cure for Alzheimer's disease. Marked by difficulty recalling recent events and storing new memories, this neurodegenerative condition typically occurs spontaneously. These cases are not linked to genetic factors, but they are linked to obesity. A just released ten year study from the *JOURNAL NEUROLOGY* shows cognitive decline in obese participants to be as much as twenty-two and one-half percent faster than for those of normal weight with no risk factors. This study is also significant in that it debunks the concept of being 'fit and fat' by demonstrating that despite apparent metabolic health, the cognitive profile was still poor.

The rare neurodegenerative cases that are genetic have been thought to travel through the female bloodline. Interestingly, bioidentical (identical in structure and function to what we make in our own body) estradiol can help prevent the loss of memory for these women as it prevents the folding of proteins, something Premarin could not do.

Escalating symptoms of Alzheimer's include a disrupted sense of time and space, irritability, mood swings, and social withdrawal. Currently, five point four million Americans suffer from this condition, thirteen percent of them over the age of sixty-five. What has been noted with interest is that patients on the blood pressure lowering drug angiotensin II receptor blockers (ARBs) cut their risk by fifty percent and they are also twenty-five percent less likely to develop vascular dementia. It is speculated that the ARB drugs cause biochemical changes in the brain, which attack the causes. Arthritis sufferers may bypass dementia for similar reasons as they typically consume lots of anti-inflammatory drugs, which have their own risks: gastrointestinal bleeding. Decreasing the size of your belly is a much safer plan of attack.

Meanwhile, all researchers are in agreement that treatment needs to start early before the brain is too severely damaged. Once again, we must consider diet and exercise to preserve what we have and forestall what may be inevitable. Good news though, you can actually be comfortably seated (and entertained!) while doing many exercises that are recommended for your brain. See www.Lumosity.com. for a fascinating array of games that will keep your brain challenged. If your future plans require your maximum brain potential for continued learning, it may be useful for you to determine Hemispheric Dominance. A test that will determine Left vs. Right and study skills help are available at http://frank.mtsu.edu/~studskl/hd/learn.html. However, before you begin spending too many more hours in front of a computer screen, keep in mind, the most recent statistics I've seen indicate that aerobic activity of one-half hour or longer three to four times weekly is most efficacious in insuring an adequate nutrient supply to the brain. A first-of-it's-kind government sponsored study is currently experimenting with Resveratrol (a natural compound found in red wine) to see if it can alter or delay the destruction of the brain in persons with mild to moderate Alzheimer's.

Dr. Daniel Amen, creator of SPECT Brain Scans, has published eighteen studies, which demonstrate that "as your weight goes up, the physical size and function of your brain goes down." This is what he calls 'Dinosaur Syndrome', big body, little brain. Dr. Amen takes issue with the conventional psychiatric treatment of brain related problems through pharmaceuticals because "there is no actual science to prove that it is useful to the patient". On the other hand, targeted treatment through diet and exercise is where his program excels in treating cases of ADD/ ADHD, depression and bipolar disorder. You can find his free brain audit at www.amenclinics.net. He has a program, The Amen Solution at home- which offers a two week trial membership for one dollar. Always amusing, Dr. Amen points out that the brain is the only organ in the body that we hadn't previously examined when we were attempting to manage it's malfunction. You can see tremendous improvements tracked through his protocol and scanning on his web site.

Dr. William L. Wilson of the CARB Syndrome Project claims that we have "scrambled our brains with sugar. It's not weight that's a problem so much as fat storage... and the brain calls the shots." One hundred years ago, we consumed one pound sugar per person annually, and now the average is one hundred-fifty pounds. Fructose is the primary driver of insulin resistance. "Combining excessive fructose with HGC is directly responsible for the increase in many chronic brain disorders including -Depression, ADHD, Autism, eating disorders, fibromyalgia, irritable bowl syndrome, PTSD, bipolar II, anxiety disorders, and others. With insulin resistance, and rapidly absorbed carbohydrate consumption, your brain is subject to toxic glucose spikes, which cause mitochondrial dysfunction leading to depletion of important neurotransmitters such as dopamine, norepinephrine, and serotonin. Initially, this leads to cravings for sweet and starchy foods- the very foods that are frying your brain, and just like a hibernating bear, you will hold on to stored fat".

For whatever reason, I find that most of my acquaintances that have these conditions are very locked into their treatments with psychiatry and pharmaceuticals. I mention that there are great doctors around now who can help them get off their meds and address these problems at their root. I mention the unknown effects of years of medications... the possible unwanted side effects. Does the pharmaceutical industry have such an awesome lobby that we dare not question this protocol? Are the symptom stabilizing effects of meds that dependable? (I don't see that to be the case!) Are the suffering victims so worried about exposing themselves and their loved ones to additional trauma that they dare not try?

If getting off ones meds is still too daunting a proposition, perhaps Professor Gary Wenk, author of the book "YOUR BRAIN ON FOOD" can help. He claims that heading off dementia begins with what we eat. Like the drugs we put into our body, food is made up of chemicals that prompt a reaction in the brain. Choosing the right foods can minimize damage and preserve a healthy mind as we age. He does an admirable job of explaining the free radical damage we experience and how we can borrow from nature's natural plant protectors, the antioxidants, as a fine hedge against dementia. He believes that consuming a wide array of antioxidant containing foods negates the need for vitamins and supplementation.

Citing **BMI** as the most accurate predictor of *lifespan*, Wenk says: "First fat ages you, then it kills you". Any baby boomer pot heads out there reading this will be happy to read this **TIP:** one 'hit' per evening of your preferred prescription can alleviate inflammation in an aging brain, according to Professor Wenk. However, if you never stop at one hit, I suggest you look online at Dr. Amen's SPECT Brain Scans of pot addicts and get a clue... Moderation anybody?

YOU'VE GOTTA HAVE HEART

"Oh Lord, help me to be pure, but not yet."
~ Saint Augustine

"We'll love you just the way you are if you're perfect."
~ Alanis Morissette

"Someday, after mastering the winds, the waves, the tides, and gravity, we shall harness for God the energies of Love, and then, for a second time in the history of the world, man will have discovered fire."
~Pierre Teilhard de Chardin

"How on earth are you ever going to explain in terms of chemistry and physics so important a biological phenomenon as first Love?"
~ Albert Einstein

Well, Dr. Einstein, I'd like to introduce you to Dr. Helen Fisher. If we could somehow time travel you to 2012, I feel certain that you and Helen would enter into some kind of Vulcan mind meld that the rest of us fools would call love...

If Helen hasn't already committed her heart elsewhere, she would know just how to massage that oversized brain of yours and turn your feet to jelly. Because, you see, Helen has all the secrets to love. Since the Garden of Eden, it seems, men have asked "how do you make love last"? Helen has the answers!

Dr. Helen Fisher is a Biological Anthropologist who has authored 5 books, including *ANATOMY OF LOVE* and *WHY WE LOVE*. She is affiliated with the matchmaking site, CHEMISTRY.com where over seven million people have taken the test, which she developed to help us all find and keep lasting love. You can also go to the Helen Fischer home page and take the test as well as share it on Facebook.

I reference Dr. Fisher's work here because I am a Pisces woman and it is said of us that we need love more than we need air to breathe. When I look at the stunningly dismal statistics on women and heart disease, I can't help but think that Pisces, being the twelfth sign, and the so called dust bin of the zodiac, simply reflects the needs of all the signs that came before it. What I'm saying here, I guess, is that we all need love; we just need it in slightly different ways. Women are generally much more in touch with their need then men, though men benefit significantly in terms of their health and longevity from being in a committed relationship.

I was very moved last year by a human-interest news story about a couple where the man had a heart attack and died instantly. His wife died of an actual broken heart shortly thereafter. Yes, broken hearts are a reality! However, broken or not, heart disease is the leading cause of death of women in the United States. Approximately five times the number of women who die of breast cancer will die from heart attacks. *That's FIVE times MORE!* What's even more stunning is that it is often not accurately diagnosed and these women do not receive the care that they need, including an analysis of their physical *inactivity*. As breast cancer is the most common type of cancer affecting women, you'll be pleased to note that a regular exercise program can reduce your risk by *thirty* percent. Also, there is promising news from scientists at Pennsylvania State College of Medicine who have discovered a virus "that is capable of killing all grades of breast cancer" and does not cause disease. God speed!

And while far too many of us here on planet Earth are still inactive, we have been witness to some very rare activity from the planet Venus, ruler of love and the heart. Venus just passed across the Sun last week, something she will not do again for one hundred twenty-one and one half years. Given the power of symbols, this is said to be re-acclimating our planet to the potential of the Divine Feminine. Known as The Morning Star, or Bringer of Light, this crossing of the Sun is said to usher in a higher level of unity in our planetary consciousness. I feel like singing the song ... "then peace will guide the planet and love will steer the stars... this is the dawning of the Age of Aquarius... *AQUARIUS!"*

Some singing would be good right now, along with lots of dancing... Many people I know have been so beaten down by the economy and the loss of homes and jobs that they don't feel entitled to much joy in their lives lately. Joy needs to be a priority again! It's a real shame that a manmade crisis where some of the very rich got much richer and the middle class has been substantially diminished can so dominate our planetary consciousness.

Yes, the heart needs joy! The heart needs love. The heart needs aerobic conditioning as well and a diet rich in the Omegas (good fats). While I have mentioned the benefits of interval training before in these pages, I haven't driven home the idea that this is a thoughtful method to safely train the organ and substantially increase endurance as well as burn tons of calories (four times as many calories each time you approach your maximum heart rate plus a speeded up metabolism for that day according to at least one study).

If you have been unable to budge in terms of weight loss and capacity for intensity in exercise, you really must find help and supervision to get you going. It is a bit uncomfortable in the beginning if you are not used to the level of exertion that will most benefit you. This is what trainers are for. This is what classes are for. This won't really happen if you limit your workout to the Pilates reformer. Come to the water girlfriend! The following **TIPS** may help you insure a healthy heart:

1) If you are not accustomed to interval training and would like to make improvements in your exercise intensity, consider purchasing a **heart rate monitor**. An online search of Polar heart rate monitors - (www.polarusa.com.) will help you pinpoint the model that will be most effective for your individual needs both in the water and out. Polar responded to my query about the best monitor for aerobic activity in the water with a recommendation that we consider FT1 or FT2 as they have coded transmitters that function best in a water environment.

2) Zona Plus (www.Zona.com.) is a small hand held isometric therapy device, which has been proven in the overall management of cardiovascular fitness. Your doctor may not be aware yet of the potential benefits of the regular 12 minute training with this device which your insurance may cover. If your care giver is suggesting medication for hypertension or high blood pressure, you might persuade them to let you try this first.

TO SLEEP: PERCHANCE TO DREAM...

"Life is something that happens
when you can't get to sleep."
~ Fran Lebowitz

"The bed is a bundle of paradoxes: we go to it
with reluctance, yet we quite it with regret;
we make up our minds overnight to leave it early,
but we make up our bodies every morning to keep it late."
~ Charles Caleb Colton

"It is a common experience that a problem
difficult at night is resolved in the morning after the
committee of sleep has worked on it."
~ John Steinbeck

"And if tonight my soul may find her peace in sleep,
and sink in good oblivion, and in the morning wake
like a new opened flower, then I have been dipped again
in God and new- created."
~ D. H. Lawrence

More and more, the jury is in on sleeping and Americans are very guilty... we are failing to deal with the facts. Lack of adequate zzzzzzzzz's is a major culprit in the 'diabesity' epidemic that plagues our nation and it is responsible for inadequate job performance, problematic relationship issues, depression and panic disorder, and a generally weakened immune system.

What may be worse, if my sources are correct, is that people actually stand around the office watering hole bragging about their lack of sleep; as though three and one half hours is an achievement of some sort! I know I'd rather be hearing: "I slept like my toddler last night, out like a light, woke up eight hours later in the exact same position, can you believe it?"

Now, many of you, the guilty, may well want to shout back at me that you would love to sleep, but you cannot. There is new hope (notice I said 'hope', and not a magic bullet?) for you- an Australian program has shown significant results in conditioning the body to perform on a regular sleep schedule. Basically, they are retraining the body because they take insomniacs who had no sleep the previous night and allow them to fall asleep at the beginning of every half hour for three minutes only and repeat this process for the next twenty-five hours. The resulting 'new habit' of quickly nodding off stays with most subjects who are tracked for the next six months. The Flinders sleep lab is considering the sale of portable sleep monitors with alarm signals as an at home remedy. If you are among the true insomniacs, you might give their system a go.

You could also try what's worked for me in the past when circumstances have found me sleepless... Make yourself stay awake until you reach the time where you should be sleeping if you were to get the requisite six to eight hours that your body craves. Sleep restriction, not over sleeping, is also an important aspect of this recalibration. This is your dedicated sleep time (even if you do not actually sleep all of the hours) and it needs to be respected and honored as mankind's mandatory astral travel and rebooting ritual.

As an accidental athlete, I was financially compelled to reinvent myself as a morning person and despite the difficulties in that transformation, the rewards are great. Either moodiness is cured in such a regular sleep process or there is just something so fresh and hopeful about the early morning hours. Supposedly, we get more bang for our buck by drinking coffee outdoors in the natural blue light of day when we *want* our melatonin levels to be suppressed. If you're a frequent traveler, getting outdoors in the midday light and doing a bit of military style marching (opposite arm and leg working in tandem) will help overcome your jet lag according to my training in applied kinesiology.

A study done at Northwestern University took sedentary adults and put them on an aerobic conditioning program four times weekly to very good effect. Not only was their sleep quality much improved, but tendencies towards depression where greatly reduced as well. The following are some general **TIPS** for improving the outcome of your sleep ritual:

1) Aerobic **exercise** is a boon to sleeping well, but it is not so helpful when done too close to the dedicated sleep hour, there's nothing like a regular and intense early morning exercise class to get you sleeping like a baby at night. If you are among the ten percent of our population that suffers from restless legs syndrome, an aquatic exercise class may be just the ticket.

2) No caffeine, no night cap, no spicy or sugary foods close to the dedicated time. What may help is an unrefined carbohydrate cereal featuring oats, corn, or rice. If you use almond milk and a not too ripe banana, you get even more of the sleep hormone, melatonin. A half turkey sandwich (bread featuring the oats or rice) will also do the trick, as can a few dried tart cherries. I also like Source Naturals Melatonin Spray, a spritz or two under the tongue will kick-in faster that a pill.

3) Make the bedroom as **dark** as possible, you may need to put some black tape over any of the stray blue lights that can suppress production of melatonin. This includes some alarm clocks, stereos, TV's, and computers. It may be better to not have some of these things in the bedroom as some people are extremely sensitive to electronic devices. I have a red bulb in my reading lamp as I read that the red ray was more beneficial and it has proven to be very helpful when I read myself to sleep.

4) The recommended **temperature** for sleeping is between fifty-four and seventy-five degrees. If cold feet keep you awake, slip on a pair of socks and you'll feel snug as your core body temperature drops, initiating sleep.

5) Statistics clearly show that a good nights sleep is not had by all when there are animals and/or children in the bed. So sorry! Sleeping with your mate however, can give some kind of primal comfort despite the fact that women wake up more often during the night than when sleeping alone. Treating relationship issues can improve insomnia. If snoring that involves gasping for air is a problem, sleep apnea is suspect and can lead to serious or fatal medical conditions when left untreated. An easy fix, do it!

6) Activities in bed may need to be restricted to sleep and sex... laptops, texting, TV's and the like may not interfere with some but if you're an insomniac, they are highly suspect.

7) Consider whether your **bedding** needs sprucing up. For myself and my clients sleeplessness can sometimes be aggravated by an old pillow that no longer offers sufficient support. After an automobile accident last year, I found that a memory foam neck pillow with a pouch and a hot/ cold insert (check Bed, Bath, and Beyond) became my most priceless possession. New items to consider are personalized comforters where couples can customize the amount of filling in each half of the comforter. Since nineteen eighty-seven, the same company (Select Comfort Corporation) has sold mattresses with adjustable firmness in each side.

8) In a pinch, both sleeplessness and stress can be greatly relieved with some focused **breathing**. Make your body as comfortable as possible in your bed first. Then beginning with your toes, point and flex, separate and wiggle, then moving up to the ankles, circle, breathing deeply all the while. Slowly move up the body (centering on Chakras if you're into Yoga) focusing on the muscle tension or pain as you flex in that area and then release it with the exhale. When you reach the neck and shoulders continue locating the tightness and releasing it with the exhale. Now feeling as relieved of body tension as possible, inhale deeply through both nostrils and then curl the right index and middle fingers into your palm and press the right nostril closed with the right thumb. Now exhale slowly and deeply through the left nostril, followed by a slow inhale. Next, use the index and middle fingers to close the left nostril and inhale through the right side...exhale slowly, then repeat with the thumb closing the right side and breathing through the left. Alternate as needed for several cycles. You may notice that one nostril feels more open than the other as dominance fluctuates throughout the day in thirty to one-hundred- twenty minute intervals. If you are having trouble falling asleep and the right side (a more yang, active energy) is dominant, then rolling onto the opposite left side will switch dominance (the yin, feminine) ... Sweet Dreams!

OUR EARTH, OUR CURE

"We do not need magic to transform our world.
We carry all the power we need inside ourselves already. "
~ JK Rowling

"Scared and Sacred are spelled with the same letters.
Awful proceeds from the same root word as awesome.
Terrify and terrific. Every negative experience holds
the seeds of transformation."
~ Alan Cohan

As I begin writing today, I feel obliged to share with you some rather yucky details of my last couple months. Fool that I can be, I broke my toe on a piece of furniture almost exactly two months ago. I went through a phase ten years past where I broke the same toe (on the opposite foot!) four times, three times on a cumbersome queen sized bed before I accepted the fact that the room itself necessitated a double bed. The fourth break happened in the water, as soon as I felt 'healed', I taught water aerobics without taping the toes together or wearing shoes and voila! "Snap", it went on my first series of big kicks. Lesson learned!

So this time, after striking a rather ridiculous claw foot, which 'graced' an early American table, I decided to be more vigilant. I taped and taped the toes together like a maniac because waterproof tape isn't always so. It drove me crazy coming off and I got lazy when I found that it stayed on best if

I just kept it taped, all the time. Finally, that strategy (denial!) resulted in inflammation and itchiness, which got me up in the middle of the night to cut off bandages and apply soothing unguents. Today, after my long spin and sculpt class, I'm treating very itchy blisters around and under three toes. I thank my lucky stars that I have enough sense to keep a glass jar of French green clay prepared for action. I keep it stored on top of my oven where there is some continuous warmth and occasionally, I place it in the sunshine and add some water if it gets too thick and appears to be drying up.

I will add a few drops of the natural antiseptic tea tree oil to a quarter cup of prepared clay and apply the paste all over between the toes and then wrap it with some old strips of t-shirt or toweling (before placing a plastic sandwich bag over it) and I will enjoy the wonderful sense of relief that comes as the paste starts to draw out all the 'itchiness'. When I lose patience with it in a half hour or so, I will remove the wrappings and allow it to dry. Then I will rinse the clay away and follow with some more tee tree oil. This cure from the Earth has been a godsend for me so many times in my life that I don't know how any household could exist without their supply of healing clay.

In my early twenties I found the book "OUR EARTH OUR CURE" by Raymond Dextreit and it saved me then when I suffered from terrible eczema, which, I believe was a result of extreme exposure to toxic substances in oil paint and turpentine... After reading the book, I applied a poultice over my liver before going to bed at night. It was recommended that you cover the 'goo' with a thin layer of onionskin or cabbage leaves before wrapping it with cloth. At any rate, when I awakened in the morning, I removed the poultice and there were many boil like blisters on the surface of my skin. I aired the skin and kept reapplying to draw out the toxins. Convinced that this was a blessing to me, I decided to do the internal liver cleanse as recommended in the book. It's a combination of a small amount of food grade clay taken orally in water for some days along with a lemon juice and olive oil blitz that is a bit disgusting but effective. If you have any condition that is defying conventional treatments (or you simply want to try a natural method), I would urge you to get the book.

On another occasion in my twenties, I was preparing a large dinner for friends when I had a little grotesque accident with the blender where the glass container broke and I nearly lost my finger. Fortunately, I had my trusty stash of French green clay powder, which I had on hand to make my poultices and facial masks. I recalled that I could use the food grade clay powder to stop bleeding and it worked miraculously! I applied pressure (squeezing the wound edges together) with clay powder thinking I'd better find a ride to the emergency room for some stitches. Soon, I was very pleasantly surprised that the bleeding was stopped. Everyday, I changed the bandages and applied a fresh clay poultice to the wound. Layers of skin kept peeling away in the final stages of healing, as there was practically no scar...

Now for those of you seeking more refined, glamorous skin, nothing seems to beat the efficacy of a green clay mask. Particularly effective after steaming the pores open... you can do the towel tent trick over a bowel of steamy hot water- if you have some fresh mint, lavender, or essential oils to add to the water, why not?

To prepare your stash of clay, I suggest a smallish glass jar with a glass lid if possible. There are some very pretty jars of that design, which were intended for food gifting. It is recommended that you add clay powder to the water (purified or mineral, please!) without stirring... it becomes much more potent if you allow the water to slowly infuse the clay on it's own without stirring. At this point, if you can set it in some strong sunshine, it becomes more potent still. Here are a few **TIPS** for tailoring treatments to your skin type:

1) Oily Skin that's prone to acne and large pores will benefit from the addition of a few drops of tea tree oil, citrus essential oils (orange, tangerine, grapefruit) or fresh lemon juice and/or the pulp scraped from the inside of an aloe vera leaf. Bottled aloe vera gel or witch hazel astringent can be used instead of water to make your clay. A dab of raw honey can be another healing addition. While you're preparing your facial mask, you might want to customize an astringent with the same ingredients (minus the clay) to apply after removing the dried mask (try to hang on for twenty minutes or longer) It's good to cover your face with a steamy (old as it will discolor) towel and help the clay soften-up for a gentle removal, so as not to aggravate the skin to more oiliness.

2) Dry, Mature Skin will benefit from the addition of moisturizing ingredients such as yogurt, raw honey, avocado, and/or the addition of a skin toner made with herbs that suite your skin type. Be aware that only a small amount of your prepared clay should be combined with these food items as it will now (unlike the pure clay) be more subject to spoilage. After gently removing and rinsing, be sure to begin moisturizing before the skin dries. Also, it is good to moisturize the eye area before the application of steam or mask.

3) Stretch Marks and Cellulite may respond to repeated applications of a paste made with clay and the addition of used coffee grounds as well as an oil such as coconut or olive. Optional drops of tee tree oil may be good as will a vigorous rubbing of the area with the paste (this requires patience as stimulating the skin to produce more collagen will not happen quickly).

4) Eggplant Skin Treatment may eliminate Actinic Keratosis with twice daily applications- blend a chunk of organic eggplant (contains solasodine glycosides) in your blender with sufficient apple cider vinegar to cover. Store in a glass jar in your refrigerator and mix a small amount with equal parts clay and apply to affected area. For more information, order *THE EGGPLANT CANCER CURE BOOK* by Dr. Bill Cham available from the Tahoma Clinic Pharmacy (www.tahomadispensary). where you can also order the prepared skin cream, BEC5 (Curaderm) and micropore tape.

5) Clay Baths are a natural way to detoxify the body when exposed to such things as excessive radiation or poison ivy. Mix 1/2 cup of clay powder in a quart of water and add it to your bath. Adding a few drops of essential oil such as lavender is a boost and/ or fresh lavender, sage, rosemary, or mint tied together or wrapped in thin cheesecloth. Relax and enjoy!

A TWENTY-ONE-DAY CHALLENGE

"Action is the antidote to despair."
~ Joan Baez

"You change for two reasons: either you learn
enough that you want to or you've
been hurt enough that you have to."
~Unknown

"Change the overall conviction that you can't do
anything and you will be able to do everything."
~ Unknown

"The 3 C's of life: choices, chances, and changes.
You must make a choice to take a chance or your life
will never change."
~Unknown

Think for just a moment how much extra 'cha ching' you might have available if you were to quite a really nasty habit such as smoking. The cash in the pocket really starts to add up. I say that not because I assumed that you smoke but rather because getting rid of other less obvious, harmful behaviors and replacing them with more healthful choices and behaviors is going to give you the 'cha ching' that you have yet to imagine...

It has been demonstrated that most any habit can be broken in twenty-one days, the first three days may be the hardest when you will need to *plan* just exactly *how* you will distract yourself from the desire to give in. After twenty-one days, the desire may still return, though less frequently, but now you will have the strength to ignore it until it passes and you will have a psychological system or a better habit in place that allows the desire to pass without suffering, and eventually without notice.

If you could use a personal trainer or a little life coaching here, maybe I can help. Why not think of the year ahead as an opportunity to make twelve lasting changes in your choices and behavior? Think of six such habits (what, *you* don't have six?) that you believe are detrimental to your health and well-being and then choose six new behaviors (as you browse this little book!) that you would like to manifest in your life.

Before you write this off as being too ambitious for a busy person like yourself, consider the following: the taste for sugar, salt, and fat are acquired habitual cravings. Going to bed too late every night and suffering the many health consequences of insufficient sleep is a habit. Planning to go to the gym and letting something 'more important' come up is a habit. Starving yourself all day and then comforting yourself with food at night is a habit. I'm certain that if you really think about it, you may come up with others that I haven't mentioned.

The important thing is to limit your agenda to just *one* habit at a time. Typically, people get too ambitious when they seek improvements in their lives. It's just too difficult to take on so much 'change' at once and the times we live in may be throwing some curve balls our way as well. So, don't set yourself up for failure, choose one!

I say you choose your nastiest behavior first, the one that gives you the most guilt or anxiety and let's get that out of the way first. After that, it's all a piece of cake (an edible bouquet to you!). Can you imagine how different your life might become twelve months from now?

In order to tackle that most nasty habit, consider whether you have the will power to break it alone or whether you require a support group. There are many such groups in large cities. You don't have to be an alcoholic to attend most AA meetings, if a drink or two is routinely ruining your plans to get healthier- find a meeting, it will give you the inspiration that will speed you on your way. The same for Overeaters Anonymous. Some of my clients here in LA will check in with Weight Watchers periodically if they feel out of control. It gives you a 'reckoning' at the weigh-in, a knowledgeable support group with convenient meeting times and understanding their point system can get you through social eating situations where temptation lurks. As for implementing a new exercise habit, an acquaintance with the same goal who lives nearby can be an invaluable asset. It can be even better if the buddy is not a really close friend as our closest friends are often partners in our bad behaviors. Sometimes it's better to make a new friend.

My suggestion? Buy a notebook and begin to do a little daily journaling. You do not need to have any writing skills to benefit from a journal; it is yours alone. Your writing can be dry as toast, or illegible to most and it will still accomplish the task- making you more accountable to yourself. It will also help you tap into your subconscious by facilitating daydreaming. During a focused endeavor such as this, we can suddenly become aware that we've outgrown some old dreams and new ones are waiting in the wings to be discovered and embraced. Further down the road, if something throws you off course temporarily, rereading parts of your journal may set you right again immediately. You can list the facts, of course; what you ate, what you did or didn't do. Even more importantly, it should include how you feel, what issues you are struggling with in the process.

When you feel the desire to give in, do not give in! Make it a point to do something *different*, drop everything and go out for a brisk walk, get to the swimming pool. Interrupt the desire with action! This can be the perfect time to spoil yourself a little bit with a soothing massage. I highly recommend a detox foot bath and infrared sauna. If support groups are not for you , or you simply lack the time to take a meeting, consider a small investment in CD's from www.hypnosisnetwork.com. They are highly recommended, affordable (compared to a heftier price tag for individual treatments), and claim to boost weight loss by more than one-hundred-forty percent.

Now there may be some readers out there who scoff at the idea that they can make that *big* change in one months time. If failure is commonplace in your life regarding that one worst nasty habit, let's go a different direction! Counterintuitively thinking, let's go for a couple of your lesser bad habits first. If, for instance, permanent weight loss is your goal but you have failed on many diets in the past, let's choose just one component for change at a time, perhaps an addiction to diet soda? Eliminating just this one item for your challenge will set you on the path towards meeting your ultimate goal.

Trying a variety of teas instead, with a stevia sweetener, will boost your health in two ways. One; they may well increase your fat burning metabolism, the polysaccharides in tea appear to have glucose inhibiting properties. According to a two-thousand-nine German study, it can reduce the expression of genes associated with new fat growth and breakdown some of the existing fat as well. If you don't care for the taste, try it in a flavored variety or mix it with a black tea variety that you like. White tea has less caffeine than black or green but a bonus in being able to slow the enzyme responsible for breakdown of elastin and collagen... a beauty bonus! I take a thermos with me on a long day away from home and pick up some ice as the day gets warmer. It's also fun to invest in a lovely tea pot and create a new ritual when friends drop in to visit. So civilized!

If you take this approach towards meeting your weight loss goals, month two could be giving up all processed packaged snack foods. Again, give it some thought and get creative. After years of burning-out my air poppers for popped corn, I bought a Whirley*poP Jr., which uses one tablespoon of oil. I've found that coconut oil and my herb salt make a snack so divine, my guests can barely control themselves! If you have an insatiable desire for something that's full of chemicals, try to locate a healthier version and then split it up into small baggie servings to be supplemented with sliced veggies, fruits, etc. (Try to keep snacks at one hundred to one-fifty calories.)

I will bet you that these two relatively simple changes in your lifestyle over a period of two months will also result in weight loss and increased enthusiasm for meeting your ultimate goal. Possibly you can continue on in this manner by channeling this enthusiasm into a new *physical* challenge for the third month. Try committing to three aquatics classes weekly (remember to write it into your schedule and do not discuss!) Additionally, try something new on the days when you cannot make it to a class. Most of my clients and relatives have invested in at least one piece of exercise equipment that sits collecting dust in the basement. New research shows that just ten minutes of exercise spaced throughout the day four times will substantially increase your caloric expenditure. Dig that equipment out of storage and put it near your television... hit it hard for ten minutes while you indulge in your guilty pleasure! Walk your dog at a good pace and wear some one pound wrist weights (need I say "nix the weights for a monster dog..."?) You can do this!

By the end of month three, your goal of permanent weight loss will begin to become reality and you never went on a diet... For your convenience, and to speed you on your way, make copies of the included WEIGHT-LOSS ACTION WORKSHEET, keep one with your journal to help you strategize your next goal, keep one in your wallet, and post one with refrigerator magnets to serve as a reminder when you open that door. If you are the proud owner of a magnificent automobile, and you know that it requires premium gas, regular servicing, and loving care, as well as driving time, you would not compromise on any one of those things. Why should the wonderful body you are privileged to inhabit get lesser treatment?

My favorite Dentist used to have the ceilings over his treatment chairs completely covered with inspirational quotes that he'd had done in beautiful calligraphy. I would be all anxious about some procedure that was in progress (sometimes silenced by a wad of gunk in my mouth, as well) and it always helped to look up and ponder the memorable words of another. You noticed I went all out with quotes at the top of this chapter? Well I can't resist a couple more as you prepare for this journey that will change your life...

"Imagination is everything.
It is the preview of life's coming attractions."

"Thought is the organizing factor in man,
intersected between the causal
primary instincts and the resulting actions.
Once we accept our limits, we go beyond them."

"The measure of intelligence is the ability to change."

~ Albert Einstein

WEIGHT-LOSS ACTION WORK-SHEET:

If you've been stuck in 'yo yo' dieting or failed attempts at permanent weight loss:

DOCTOR CONSULTATION:

1) Permission to exercise vigorously in water- interval training and rebounding aerobics. If 'moderate only' exercise is recommended, what modifications need to be made?
2) The ALCOT test & 24 hour urine test reveal *allergies, sensitivities, and deficiencies-*
3) Do my metabolic issues allow for 10 to 30 minutes of exercise before breakfast?

21-DAY CHALLENGE PLAN: What 'addictive' tastes and behaviors impede progress? Address these *1 at a time*, beginning on the 1st of each month, *plan* my next challenge during week 4 of this month & ascertain changes noticed due to *actions* taken. **KEEP A JOURNAL-** prevent backsliding, affirm success, strengthen conviction- *you can do this!*

1) If **exercise** as a consistent priority is a past failure, here's **challenge 1:** 6 days weekly, 40 to 60 minutes... 2-3 classes weekly at your pool, especially if weight and/ or joint issues prohibit vigorous land based exercise. Non-negotiable, do not discuss! On busy days, break it up - 3 or 4 units of 10 to 30 minutes. If *intensity* eludes you, try a heart rate monitor. Aerobic activity burns calories, but also aim to increase muscle mass; water exercise can accomplish both!

2) Consider a food **'addiction'** for the next challenge. If it's *sugar*, recognize the biological similarity to alcohol addiction and plan for alternative beverages and foods. HFCS and artificial sweeteners need to go! Other taste 'addictions' include packaged, processed, salty, fatty foods and refined carbohydrates. New wisdom say's it's not just calories, but *kind* of calories. A support group or **www.hypnosisnetwork.com** can be helpful.

3) Perfect fitting jeans worn weekly can be a stimulus to **portion control**. However, if your **BMI** is greater than 30, your Doctor has you *jumping* on a scale. Don't overdo that 'exercise' if it discourages you. In EXTREME REMEDIES, learn Susan's **TRICKS** such as a *weekly* calorie count, utilizing tools available at **www.lifesizeportions.com**, and **www.myfitnesspal.com** as well as her **RULES.** Armed with information, you can beat this *without* surgery. Susan say's "I have to do the work *anyway!*"

4) *FUN* challenges: up your veggie quotient to 5-10 servings daily (get a free wallet card featuring the 'dirty dozen' and 'consistently clean' at **www.foodnews.org).** Try fresh veggie juices made to order & google most any recipe to find a healthier version- Tea rituals are a great way to include friends, enlist support with *lifestyle upgrades.*

5) Find a fitness pal? This interaction can help solidify new habits... consider a trainer! Online newsletters to inspire- **www.drhyman.com, www.thehealthyeatingsite.com**

AGING GRACEFULLY?

"Old age ain't no place for sissies."
~ Henry Lewis Menckin

" Middle age is when you're old enough to know better but still young enough to do it."
~ Unknown

"Thirty-five is when you finally get your head together and your body starts falling apart."
~ Caryn Leschen

"Forty is the old age of youth, fifty is the youth of old age."
~ Victor Hugo

"What most persons consider as virtue, after the age of 40 is simply a loss of energy."
~ Voltaire

"To be seventy years old is sometimes far more cheerful and hopeful than to be forty years old."
~ Oliver Wendell Holmes JR

"Age is opportunity no less than youth itself."
~ Henry Wadsworth Longfellow

There are many arguments to be made for living a long life... but wait, that would have to be a long, healthy life, or rather, a long, healthy, happy, and prosperous life. I guess I've read too much science fiction to be easily persuaded, though I grant you, there are no good alternatives. Science fiction writer Robert Anson Heinlein's famously recurring character Lazarus Long was born in nineteen-twelve and lives approximately two thousand years. As the oldest (fictional) member of the human race, he is considered a 'mutation' in an experiment that was meant to increase his lifespan to one hundred-fifty or even two hundred years. He must, at times, lie about his age and keep moving to avoid unwanted scrutiny, disbelief, and probably overdue taxes with unimagined penalties.

When I have a little more leisure time, I know I will enjoy revisiting Heinlein's body of work and savoring the humor and irony which no doubt inform the life of the long-lived Long. I remember our mandatory reading of Heinlein's *STRANGER IN A STRANGE LAND* in high school and being swept away with the idea that we were in the midst of a great cultural shift, my generation was gonna get with the 'grock' and manifest a different reality here on planet Earth. It can be so very disappointing to realize that change generally happens slowly.

At the age of eighteen, I heard an audiotape of Baba Ram Dass (formerly Richard Alpert, professor at Harvard University who famously researched the nature of consciousness with Timothy Leary, Aldous Huxley, Allen Ginsberg and others). I clearly remember him speaking of the *PLAYBOY PLAYMATE OF THE MONTH* and saying that all the while she's being celebrated for holding this title -- she is simultaneously wondering "Is this it... Is this all there is?"

As a female living most of her adult life in a city that is notoriously unfriendly to aging women, I have to laugh when I consider that I've been made to feel 'old' since my late twenties. I felt compelled to comply with the notion that I was indeed 'old' and yet all the while, despite being an 'old soul', I have secretly felt so very young. Having grown up with a bevy of very strong and long-lived females, I now understand that I succumbed to a cultural bias that is in direct opposition to my genetic gift. My father's mother, my Mema, was candid in her bragging, "people in our family don't start to get old 'til they hit fifty."

I now understand that there are two 'flaws', if you will (keep your sense of humor here!), in the human design. One is the weakness in the skeletal system at the low back, and the other is in the hormonal system that starts to shut down; usually at about fifty, give or take some years. These days, we trainers address our skeletal vulnerability with an emphasis on core training. Aside from looking youthful, a slim and muscular core will do wonders to keep you in the game of life (not to mention games of sport!). There is really nothing quite like vertical exercise in water for enjoyably and effectively challenging the core. As for hormonal balance, some may want to argue with me that menopause or peri-menopause is not actually an estrogen deficiency disease just as andropause is not actually a testosterone deficiency disease. However, disease or not, deficiency or not, the means to safely extend the prime of life is available now and there are many wonderful board certified anti-aging doctors available to assist you in learning to use bioidentical hormone replacement. Someday, and perhaps sooner than I can imagine, the genetic keys will be utilized to prompt our bodies to continue manufacturing our own balanced hormones. For now, I encourage young women to get your hormone levels checked in your prime (late twenties to mid thirties), when you're feeling really good, so that you will know later on what levels you want to approximate with bioidenticals or genetic tweaking (should you be so lucky!).

It's irritating to me that we now see commercials on TV for testosterone supplementation for men as well as erectile dysfunction meds. (I'm not really guilty of penis envy here, as men are not being considered for a full spectrum of hormones either.) For women, all I've seen is anti-depressants being re-marketed as a 'cure' for PMS and/or menopause. We can all thank the Goddess/ Suzanne Summers and look for her books:*THE SEXY YEARS, AGELESS, BREAKTHROUGH, KNOCKOUT, BOMBSHELL,* etc. It is critical that we educate ourselves about our hormonal system, alternative health treatments and the terrific doctors utilizing them effectively if we want to thoroughly enjoy the many years from Queen to Krone. She interviews some of the finest doctors and other authorities and gives you their contact information.

Any of you reading this who happen to be young women, don't buy into the ageist propaganda as I did. We live in a time where you can now bank your eggs if having children is a priority to you. Stay fit, and you can become a mom when you're ready. For young women and men alike, if you can afford it, bank your own stem cells and you will have a most valuable resource to call upon should you later become ill.

As for the Centenarians, a fun online search will bring up pictures of many documented elders who pass the hundred mark and go as far as one hundred-twenty years. Do you see any obese people there? Not a one! In general, these folks are up-beat and happy to be alive. Most interviewers kindly agree that there is a tendency to tell the same stories repeatedly and to call the present company by the names of the long departed. They are, by necessity, good at making new friends, and the fact that they might confuse you with some long-departed friend or relative should be flattering to the youngsters who keep them company. If they never enjoyed a previous 15 minutes of fame, this is yet another chance to bask in the limelight. Otherwise, feeling that you have relevance could become a very real problem. Actually having some could be still more difficult. Especially when we consider the millions of the baby boomer silver tsunami who will shortly be putting unprecedented demands on the healthcare system. If you are among the lucky one percent who can afford the very best doctors, an exceptional diet and exercise program, as well as the cutting-edge treatments and supplements, you have the very real possibility of enjoying these years and remaining quite relevant.

Professor Wenk, whom I mentioned in the "BRAINSTORM" chapter, has studied restricted diet followers who are actually attempting to lengthen their lifespans by cutting down their caloric intake drastically. This, in an effort to eliminate as much oxidation and inflammation as possible. Followers claim that most long-lived peoples did not have particularly active lifestyles and on such a calorie restricted diet, one really couldn't. After sometime on such a diet, there is a tendency toward frailty and possible osteoporosis.

I personally don't agree with the assessment of our long-lived ancestors as being 'not particularly active'. In observing and assisting my great grandparents, I've seen the elimination of many daily chores that were previously a necessity for the average family. The simple tasks of washing and hanging out the laundry, preparing meals and cleaning up the mess were very time consuming physical labor... not to mention the chores of farm life and the rigors that attended various seasons of the year, planting crops, preserving foods, chopping wood, preparing a bath. In fact, it's my opinion that life was *harsh* for most of our ancestors. There were very good reasons why the average lifespan increased so dramatically in the twentieth century.

According to Dr. William Andrews, a biotech researcher, and expert on aging, it is the length of our Telomeres that determines how well our cells reproduce. Telomeres, which are the end-points of each chromosome, have been compared to the plastic tips on the ends of shoelaces, and they act similarly by preventing the chromosome from 'fraying'. Typically, they get shorter each time the cell divides until they become too short to divide. According to Dr.Andrews, (who also believes in taking supplements, one of which is TA-65, available at www.tasciences.com) *intense* exercise is the best way to maintain the length of telomeres and naturally extend the vitality of our middle years. Exercise, antioxidants, as well as other supplements (see the chapter SUPPLEMENT THIS!) and a positive attitude are the critical elements. Controlling our response to *stress* is essential. In an online interview offered by THE FUTURE OF HEALTH NOW, he sites an interesting study of caretakers of Alzheimer's patients, noting that their Telomeres became significantly shorter as the care-taking progressed. I mention this because so many of my favorite aquatic exercise class members are caretakers and I feel a responsibility to advocate for them. Caretakers everywhere, please eliminate guilt from your daily round and write into your schedule as *non*-negotiable the time required for you to exercise and maintain your own health and sanity!

For myself, barring accidents, I feel hopeful that I can look forward to many more healthy, active, sexy, and creative years. Part of my enjoyment of those years will be delicious meals shared with friends and relatives as well as the pleasures and challenges of physical activity in groups and solo. I'm dreaming lately of bicycling trips in France or Italy where I will really revile in the countryside, the cuisine, a little vino, and the brain stimulation of adapting to another culture and language. In these daydreams, we are peddling our way to a spa destination... of course! Wherever I may find myself living in future, I will be certain to make the location of *my* swimming pool a priority as regular water exercise will always be an integral part of my fitness and metabolic conditioning program. I understand that fighting inflammation is crucial to this plan as well as bioidentical hormone restoration and a superior diet featuring the bounty of the plant world so rich in phytonutrients. Stress management is another component to this enjoyment and not easily conquered living in a large city with lots of necessary driving, business, and monetary concerns. Certain dietary supplements are very helpful to me in this respect. In purchasing this book, *you*, dear reader, are helping me -- as I hope to engage in a more fruitful use of my time than what I've done in chasing down the almighty dollar.

In the end, I think any sane, healthy person would like to feel that their life had meaning; that they contributed somehow to the welfare of others while here or made some lasting contribution to benefit future generations. Here and now, those concerns may be instrumental to the very survival of the human race. As for the "don't worry, be happy" philosophy most of us would long to adopt, it might make you smile to know that recent research shows that when you worry (mind you, not obsess!) about your health, you are much more likely to live longer. Reason being, it mobilizes you to take positive *actions*. In the book, *THE LONGEVITY PROJECT* by Michael Freedman, he claims that the number one predictor of longevity is your ability to follow through when you say you are going to do something. After all is said and done, it's not so important how much time we spend in this life here on planet Earth as it is how we spend the time we have... In the words of funny guy Steven Wright, "I plan to live forever... so far, so good!"

A FIT PHILOSOPHY

"I no longer work for anything
but the sensation I have while working."
~ Albert Giacometti

"The only disability in life is a bad attitude."
~ Scott Hamilton

"Hurried and worried until we're buried,
and there's no curtain call,
life's a very funny proposition after all."
~ George M. Cohan

"To be successful, you have to be selfish,
or else you never achieve. And once
you get to your highest level, then you have
to be unselfish. Stay reachable.
Stay in touch. Don't isolate."
~ Michael Jordan

My Mom introduced me to Astrology as a young girl, just like she introduced me to Psychology and the world of modern medicine and its miracle drugs, which were a 'perk' in her nursing career. Of course, her interest then, like most, was in sun signs and compatibilities, but for me, it's been a life long study that has served me well in all my endeavors and dealings with others. (For free information and regular news check www.astrograph.com, www.astrologyzone.com, www.astrodienst.com, and www.spiritlibrary.com.) 'The stars do not predict, they incline...' is a favorite astrological concept and since this little book will be hitting the market soon, I must share with you my excitement that this is *it*, the much prophesied year *TWENTY-TWELVE!*

The optimistic Astrologers I like to follow suggest that rather than an ending as many believe was predicted by the ancient Mayan and Hopi Indians, this period is better viewed as a new beginning here on planet Earth. Perhaps the reason the ancients couldn't see man doing business as usual after December twenty-one was because most all mankind (or at least a critical mass!) will be vibrating at a slightly higher spiritual frequency. It has been said that when a psychic 'pierces the veil' to try and give you a peek into your future, what they 'see' and make sense of is ultimately dependent on their own experiences.

One recent issue of *THE MOUNTAIN ASTROLOGER* put it quite succinctly when an article referred to this period on Earth as 'a crisis in ethics'. That's most definitely the short story! What we do know for certain is that our little planet is supporting the largest number of human inhabitants in the history of the world, many of them starving and yet brutalized by tyrants. Meanwhile, the billions of us here now are dangerously close to destroying the precious resources, which we must have to survive.

Perhaps the late George Carlin was correct in his cutting commentary that "Man doesn't need to worry about Nature because Nature can take care of herself... she'll just shake us off like a bad case of fleas." George could make me laugh like nobodies business, but am I wrong in guessing he was, at times, a very angry man? I can relate... forget about fleas, it's the demise of bee's that's got my panties in a bunch! Initially, I set out to write a humorous fitness book that is still reality based. Laughter is, after all, a most critical element to our health and happiness. However, most of the latest research yielded up statistics and conclusions that were decidedly unfunny.

There is, however, some very encouraging information to share about us so called "CULTURAL CREATIVES". You may recall that this group constitutes America's (and the global) practical idealists...the demographics cover a very wide range of social class positions from working class to the elite. It is almost meaningless to try and describe this group in terms of occupation, education, or income, but the key identifiers are *values,* worldview, and lifestyle. While typically, these individuals experienced a sense of isolation growing up—and in fact constituted only two percent of the population in the nineteen-fifties, they now make up nearly forty percent, or more, of the American population, (two-thousand-twelve) and worldwide, continue expanding their numbers. For more encouraging information, check out www.wisdomuniversity.org/emerging-culture.htm. Many on our planet seem to believe that the old world is dying at the hands of an angry God. The emerging wisdom holds that something newer and more fundamentally humane is arising in it's place. "We are transitioning from an era of change to a change of eras." On those days when you might feel down, it really helps to know that *shift* can happen.

For the real deal on the current astronomical realities, see *2012 - THE REAL STORY* a lecture by Lee Carroll at www.KRYON.com. Lee does a magnificent job explaining some very complex ideas to people like me. Apparently December twenty-one marks the mid-point of a *thirty-six* year period of accelerated change featuring "the highest potential for expanding human consciousness that Earth has ever seen". According to Lee, the media has been quite biased in presenting the most frightening scenarios for these times and thus far ignoring much of what could help us navigate the wave and maximize the opportunity...

It seems to me that our best hope during these tumultuous times is in showing up as our fittest selves. We need the strength and fortitude to be able to reconnect to Nature and establish a more harmonious relationship based on respect rather than exploitation. We need to come together, acting in partnership, and take concerted actions as the stewards who tend this garden. We also need to keep our sense of humor intact as we struggle to maintain tolerance and compassion in the face of the dwindling 'pirate' mentality that has thus far been the dominant force in shaping our civilization.

Just as the research of Dr. Masaru Emoto has demonstrated previously unknown and miraculous abilities of water, scientific breakthroughs in curing cancer and all the degenerative and genetically linked diseases are ongoing realities. However, it makes sense that the resulting cures will likely work best on a body and mind that has previously been conditioned to it's optimal level of fitness. What is needed is a real and permanent lifestyle upgrade for many of us right now and a recognition that our friends, family, and even the strangers we meet in our daily round are struggling with a multitude of issues. We have the power and the responsibility to overcome our divisiveness and partisanship, and participate in a much needed global upgrade.

It is my greatest hope that you will have been informed, entertained, and inspired by some things in these pages. That you will become passionate about water exercise for yourself and others as a means to enhance your health, maintain your optimal weight, as well as manage your stress and pain. Perhaps somewhere in this little book, there will be something just for you alone, a key that will help you take the next step towards becoming the person you've always secretly believed you were meant to be. Some closing words from the accidental athlete who has aspired here to become your personal trainer and fitness coach? Love more, fear less, *love more fearlessly!*

With Appreciation and Gratitude,
~ Janna Lowell

"If God creates a world of particles and waves, dancing in obedience to mathematical and physical laws, who are we to say that he cannot make use of those laws to cover the surface of a small planet with living creatures."
~ Martin Gardner

"Everyone thinks of changing the world
but no one thinks of changing himself."
~ Leo Tolstoy

"They always say time changes things
but you actually have to change them yourself."
~ Andy Warhol

"Life shrinks and expands in proportion to one's courage."
~ Anais Nin

"I get up every morning determined to both change the world and have one hell of a good time. Sometimes, that makes planning my day difficult."
~ E. B. White

"Turbulence is life force. It is opportunity.
Let's love turbulence and use it for change."
~ Ramsay Clark

"Commit to be fit!"
~Unknown

DEDICATION

To Louise Fitzgerald who showed up for class as regularly as I but began water exercise many years before I was ever on the scene. Louise taught me things I hadn't learned in my aquatic training just as she taught her classroom students much more than their ABC's. A member of 'The Greatest Generation', she kissed her new young husband 'goodbye' as he went off to war and never saw him again. She survived two (or was it three?) additional husbands and devoted herself to charitable works. 'Til the age of eighty-five, she sported a bright and flattering swimsuit on her trim figure with matching earrings. Best of all, she was always prepared to deliver a funny joke and give us a giggle (some more naughty than you'd ever anticipate from this lady!) She was a sunny Aires, always anticipating community and church events, sometimes offering a new recipe or a recommendation to an exotic local garden. Always an inspiration, Louise made class time fly by... God Bless!

INDEX

D

I

J

K

L

M